Quit Alcohol (for a month)

Quit Alcohol
(for a month)

HELEN FOSTER

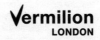
Vermilion
LONDON

1 3 5 7 9 10 8 6 4 2

Vermilion, an imprint of Ebury Publishing,
20 Vauxhall Bridge Road,
London SW1V 2SA

Vermilion is part of the Penguin Random House group of companies
whose addresses can be found at global.penguinrandomhouse.com

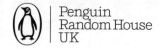

Penguin
Random House
UK

First published in the United Kingdom by Vermilion in 2017

www.penguin.co.uk

A CIP catalogue record for this book is available from the British Library

ISBN 9781785041389

Typeset in India by Integra Software Services Pvt. Ltd, Pondicherry

Printed and bound in Great Britain by Clays Ltd, St Ives PLC

Penguin Random House is committed to a sustainable future for our
business, our readers and our planet. This book is made from
Forest Stewardship Council® certified paper.

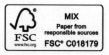

MIX
Paper from
responsible sources
FSC® C018179

The information in this book has been compiled by way of general guidance in rela-
tion to the specific subjects addressed, but it is not a substitute and not to be relied
on for medical, healthcare, pharmaceutical or other professional advice on specific
circumstances and in specific locations. Please consult your GP before changing, stopping or starting any medical treatment. So far as the author is aware the information
given is correct and up to date as at August 2017. Practice, laws and regulations all
change, and the reader should obtain up to date professional advice on any such issue.
The author and the publishers disclaim, as far as the law allows, any liability arising
directly or indirectly from the use, misuse, of the information contained in this book.

Contents

Introduction

30 days hath September

April, June and November

All the rest have 31

Except for Dry January

Which has 5,782

(Tweet by @oconnola, 4th January 2016)

At some point in the next 12 months a few million people in the UK and around the world will all pledge to do the same thing – give up alcohol for the period of a month. Some will be doing it to raise money for charity, others want to improve their health or lose weight, some might even be doing it simply to test whether they can – but pretty much everyone at some point during their month-long quest utters something along the lines of the phrase 'I could murder a drink'. If that sounds like you, this is the book that aims to help stop you drinking it.

Technically, taking a month off should be easy – alcohol isn't like air, food or water. It's not something we need to physically survive. In the majority of cases, we can pick or choose whether to consume it and, considering the miserable side effects that occur if you overdo it, giving it up for what's a tiny fraction of your life should be a breeze – but often it isn't. We live in a very drinky culture here in the UK. It's almost expected of us to drink at work, at play, at celebrations and as a way to destress – say you don't drink and people often look at you with vague suspicion. Going to the pub is a major British pastime – we have over 50,000 around the country to choose from[1] and it's estimated that the average person spends a year of their life in one[2]. Drinking at home is also becoming a norm. One pound in every £10 spent in supermarkets is spent on alcohol[3].

Quitting can be tricky. There are hurdles everywhere. You've got to break a habit, you've got to use willpower, you may have to fight peer pressure, and you need to find something different to do on a Saturday night rather than simply wander down to the local. Go into a month of abstinence unprepared and you could have a pint in your hand before you can say 'I'm not drinking right now,' or spend the whole 30 days feeling grumpy, deprived and miserable. Plan for what you're going to do though and it's far easier. You'll resist temptation, saying no will be a breeze, and you'll end the month as clinging firmly to the wagon as you were when you started. The job of this book is to help you organise that plan and find the 'alcohol-free' approach that works best for you. This combination will ensure your month off will only-feel like it lasts 5,782 days if you keep it going that long!

But what you can take from this book doesn't just stop at the end of the month; it also explores how to keep up a sensible relationship with alcohol over the long term as well. Nor does it cover only booze: you'll also find advice on how to make other changes including eating more healthily, finding time (and enthusiasm) for exercise and losing weight. Some of these changes might follow on from benefits that start during your month off; others are things you might decide to tackle afterwards because you've developed a newfound confidence in your ability to make changes. You see, when it comes to change, success begets success. As you successfully make changes in your drinking habits, your self-belief in making other changes also increases – by this time you next year you could be drinking sensibly, eating sensibly, saving cash and being stress-free (yes, you're holding a miracle cure in your hands right now!). But before we get to all of that though, let's just explore the idea of the 'alcohol-free month' ... Where on earth did the idea come from?

A Brief History of Abstinence

As a concept it's not new. There are reports from Finland in 1942 of an idea called Drip-Free January which asked people to abstain for the month as part of the war effort. Many people give up alcohol for Lent and Australia's Ocsober, campaign which asks people to give up booze for 28 of the 31 days of October, was first launched in 2008. It's generally accepted that the first 'official' campaigns in the

UK were launched in January 2013 and for this, we mostly have to thank one woman.

Her name was Emily Robinson and in 2011 she decided to give up alcohol for the month of January to help the training she was doing to run a half marathon in the February. By January 2012, Emily was working for the charity Alcohol Concern and when she decided to repeat her month off, people got interested, some joined in and the charity realised this was actually a great idea to help people reassess their drinking habits. In May 2012, Alcohol Concern announced that January 2013 would be the first official 'Dry January' in the UK. Over 4,350 people took part[4]. But in the way that two similar great ideas often appear together, British charity Cancer Research UK *also* started their own alcohol-free month off in January 2013 – this one called Dryathlon. It was so popular it raised £4 million for cancer research[5]. One year, two campaigns, lots of non-existent hangovers and from this point on, the trend just grew and grew.

Fast forward to 2016 and figures from one YouGov survey found 16 per cent of people surveyed made some attempt to quit booze during January that year[6], and during that same month, the £1 in every £10 normally spent on alcohol in British supermarkets fell to an estimated 46p[7]. Quitting is also no longer confined just to January. Other booze-free months have launched in September and October and they're also incredibly popular – the 2016 Macmillan Cancer Support campaign Go Sober for October, for example, saw over 68,000 'Soberheroes' signed up for the challenge[8].

It's also now global. People in 94 different countries signed up to the UK's Dry January campaign in 2016[9], but local events are also rapidly springing up around the world. Australia now has three different months of the year when they encourage quitting for different causes, New Zealand has a Dry July, Canada officially launched Dry Feb in 2016 with 700 people taking part, while around 16 per cent of the population happily join in Finland's version of Dry January.

The idea of all these months is simple – to give us a break from alcohol and hopefully help us reassess how much we drink. Alcohol consumption in many countries is a bit of a concern. It's been estimated that across the UK we drink almost 15,000 pints of beer and 14,000 glasses of wine every 60 seconds[10]. On average we're drinking 65 per cent more than we did in the 1960s[11]. Nearly half of all middle-aged British men are classed as drinking at levels that might damage their health, consuming on average 16 pints of beer a week each, which is two-and-half the recommended alcohol limit[12]. Women aren't faring much better – their issue is drinking at home with a glass of wine (or three) after work or once the kids are in bed. This doesn't feel like problem drinking, but in fact, the constant, drip, drip, drip of alcohol it provides to the liver can be as harmful as a one-off binge – if not more so. The net result is that June 2015 figures showed hospital admissions related to alcohol grew three times more quickly in women than men[13]. Overall, the population in the UK drinks regularly and it drinks a lot, only 15 per cent of British men and 21 per cent of women say they haven't drunk at all in a year[14], and our health is suffering because of it. Alcohol is now the third leading preventable cause of ill health in Europe[15]. At least seven different types of cancer are linked to alcohol intake and then there're all the accidents people have while under the influence. No wonder the experts would like us to take a bit of a break now and again.

There's Strength in Numbers

Of course you can quit at any time – start your own No-Booze-Vember or Alcohol-Free August, but there're some definite benefits of doing it as part of one of the organised campaigns, particularly now they are so popular. Quit during Dry January or Sober October and you won't be alone and people are less likely to be surprised when you order a soda water instead your normal tipple of choice. You might not even need to order water. Pubs and restaurants realise that millions of people are trying these campaigns – and not all of them want to stay home and rearrange the furniture while they abstain – so some are stepping up to the mark to join in. Come January particularly, mixologists at various bars get creative, adding special Mocktails to their menus. Pubs increase their orders of alcohol-free beers and magazines and newspapers run entire articles on all the different soft drinks you can consume instead of your nightly glass of wine. Fact is, it's never been as cool to quit.

So Who Am I?

Now some of you might be asking what my credentials to be your booze-free buddy for the month are? Well if you ask some of my Facebook friends, they'd say I'm the least likely person to be able to help (some even laughed when I told them what I was writing about). Frankly, I am known for spending quite a lot of time in the pub. And virtually all my posts on holiday come from a bar where something fun is happening. On top of that, I'm a journalist, and we practically bleed wine.

But my online image doesn't show the whole story – just because I'm in the pub it doesn't mean I'm consuming booze. One of my closest friends still mentions how I tricked him for years when we went dancing by buying plain tonic water while he thought I was on the G&Ts. Yes, if you see me in the pub, I am likely to have a glass of wine in front of me – but what you might not notice is that there's also a glass of ice by my side and every few sips another cube goes in. By the end of the glass 90 per cent of my drink is not vino, but melted ice. If I'm out for dinner, watch carefully and you'll notice me asking the waiter to fill my wine glass with water rather than putting it in my water glass. As such, my wine glass never looks empty – but nor is it brimming with Sav Blanc as people often assume! Don't get me wrong, I'm not a saint. Hangovers still happen, but when I want to be sensible, I'm actually very good at it. Of course, the theme of this book is not cutting back but stopping completely for a month, and over the last few years I've done that too – more than once.

I've been paid to do it for work – I had to write an article on how to quit drinking and keep your social life. I quit another time when I was running a half-marathon and I wanted to see if it helped knock any minutes off my time!

Once was just for fun. I had lived in Australia, lots of my Aussie friends were trying it and so I carried out an OcSober just to see if I could do it – I lasted a month and half. I abstained again when I was going to have my knee operated on as I wanted my liver in the healthiest state possible so I recovered quickly from the anaesthetic. And then I spent 18 months suffering from symptoms that doctors thought was caused by acid reflux – each new one I saw told me to stop drinking if I wanted to get better so I did (NB: I didn't have reflux and quitting didn't help or I'd still be abstinent). I also had quite a few weeks off while writing this book just so I could remember what worked for me – and what didn't.

Every time I've done it, I've clearly seen benefits. But despite that it's not always a breeze. After three pints of water on a night out, I'm normally desperate for a beer to break the boredom! And I admit, I have turned down events during my month off because I couldn't face struggling through a long night solely on the soda. But temporarily quitting so many times has revealed tactics that work and also what strains temptation to its limits. Between this personal experience, a whole load of tips from friends who have also completed various month free campaigns and more than 20 years' journalistic experience writing health features on how to break habits and successfully form new ones, I've collected enough advice in this area to make me a pretty good 'booze-free buddy'. I know what the hurdles are, where the pitfalls lie, I know how to fight a craving – and why willpower is not the key to most people's success. As for ways to moderate your drinking when the month is over to keep within your limits, I'm a genius (even if I do say so myself).

So without further ado, let's get started with something positive. Every psychologist I've ever spoken to has said if you want to succeed at a task, the first thing you need to do is know why you're doing it and what the benefits are going to be if you succeed. And when it comes to quitting booze – even for just one month – there are an awful lot of positives to discuss.

Months Off Around the World

January

Dry January – UK. Run by the charity Alcohol Concern, it started raising money for purely alcohol-related issues but now raises money for over 12,000 different charities. Alcoholconcern.org/dryjanuary

Tipaton Tammikuu – is the Finnish version of Dry January encouraging people to abstain for the first month of the year.

Sober Start – UK – raises money for LGBT drug and alcohol services. londonfriend.org.uk

February

Feb Fast – Australia. Quit for the shortest month. Money raised goes to youth projects around Australia. Febfast. org.au

Dry Feb – Canada: Officially launched in 2016 it's linked to the Canadian Cancer Society. Dryfeb.ca

July

Dry July – Australia. Raises money for various cancer charities around the country. The 2016 campaign saw 16,787 people sign up. Dryjuly.com

Dry July – New Zealand. Raises money for cancer services in hospitals and non-profit organisations around the country. Dryjuly.co.nz

September

Dryathlon – UK. Cancer Research UK now organise Dryathlon twice a year – January and September. The September initiative launched in 2015 and aims to give people a break after boozy summers. dryathlon.org

October

Go Sober this October – UK. Raises money for MacMillan Cancer Research. gosober.org.uk

Ocsober – Australia. Raises money for the charity Life Education which raises funds for children affected by alcohol abuse. Ocsober.com.au

CHAPTER ONE

The Benefits of Quitting

For most of us, drinking alcohol is a pleasant experience. You have a glass of wine or a pint of beer and enjoy the taste, you enjoy the company you're consuming it with and, let's be honest the effects of one or two glasses are quite nice too – that's one reason why staying off alcohol, even for just a month can be tricky: it's taking away something that gives us pleasure.

Reading this chapter is the first stage in changing that and ensuring a successful month off. When it comes to making any change in life, particularly stopping something that we enjoy, the number one way to stay motivated is to list the benefits you're going to get from altering your habits – but to do that you have to know what they are. Thankfully, alcohol is of interest to scientists and so a lot of people have investigated this for you.

Notably, in 2013 a group of 10 curious journalists working on the UK's *New Scientist* magazine decided to give up drinking for a month and scientifically measure the impact on their body[16]. They enticed some willing doctors at University College London Medical School and London's

Royal Free Hospital on board, the doctors made a series of baseline measurements and the journalists set off on their challenge. At the end of the month the volunteers had lost weight, their cholesterol had fallen and their livers were in a far healthier state than before the month begun.

Amazed, the researchers decided to repeat the experiment with more people[17]. This time the group of 10 people expanded to 104 men and women in their forties who had decided to abstain from alcohol during January. On average, before the trial, the women had been drinking 29 units of alcohol a week (nearly three bottles of wine or 14 pints of lager) and the men had been drinking 31 units, enough to class both groups as heavy drinkers. But within four weeks of abstaining, their livers had started to repair themselves and other measures of health including blood pressure and their sensitivity to the hormone insulin improved, plus they also experienced some clear short-term physical benefits like better sleep and concentration.

Hearing this might be enough for some of you to commit to your challenge right here, right now but if you need more detail read on – I'm about to discuss in detail the six main areas – and the myriad of benefits – that will change if you give up alcohol for a month.

Quitting and your Health

While it's true that in small doses alcohol can confer some health benefits, drink more than the suggested sensible amounts and alcohol's effects on the body are quite nega-tive. Abstaining is therefore rather like sending your body on a holiday, giving it a break from something that stresses it out. As such, within a matter of days of giving it up you will start to feel some clear positive benefits.

Your sleep and energy improve

This was noted by people in both of the aforementioned scientific trials, with the experts analysing that abstinence improved people's sleep by 10 per cent. The reason is simple – alcohol negatively affects your sleep. Not at first, at first it actually acts as a mild sedative causing you to drop off very quickly – this is why many people use alcohol as a nightcap. However, once you've fallen asleep everything changes. Firstly, alcohol stops you progressing through the stages of sleep in the same way as you would normally and this automatically leads to more disrupted sleep in the second half of the night. On top of this, scientists in Australia have found that your brain waves actually alter during post-alcohol sleep[18]. Instead of just producing the sedative delta waves associated with sleep and restoration, the brain also produces alpha waves not normally seen when we drop off. The researchers say this dual-wave activity confuses the brain and leads to a less restorative nights' rest – the result is that even if you sleep through the night you're more likely to experience daytime drowsiness, headaches and low mood the day after.

But it's unlikely you *will* sleep through the night. You see, normally urine production shuts down at night to allow us to sleep uninterrupted, but alcohol is a diuretic and reverses this process meaning you're more likely to need to get up to use the bathroom. Alcohol also encourages us to snore by relaxing the tissues of the throat which then vibrate as we inhale – and if there's one thing guaranteed to wake you up, it's the digging elbow of a partner who can't sleep because you're keeping them awake. Sleepwalking and nightmares are also more likely if you've been drinking.

Stop drinking and this changes almost immediately, as such, for most casual drinkers, improved sleep – and the knock-on effect of increased energy that comes with it – are the first benefits you'll notice as part of your month off.

Your liver regenerates

While changes in sleep and energy are clear physical symptoms you can feel, things are also changing inside your body at a cellular level when you quit. These aren't as easy for you to spot yourself, but rest assured they are happening – particularly in your liver.

The liver is the main organ of the body that processes alcohol. One potential danger of excessive drinking is a build-up of fat that can develop in the liver as it does this. These fat cells then secrete inflammatory compounds, which can damage the cells around them. Alcohol also damages the lining of the intestine, allowing gut bacteria to enter the bloodstream – if these reach the liver they also have the potential to damage the cells. Over time, both these types of damage can lead to scarring in the liver that at first is reversible, but if you keep assaulting the area you will develop a permanent scarring of the liver that starts to affect its function – a condition known as cirrhosis.

The risk of fatty liver increases for men if they consume more than eight units a day for two to three weeks, for women it takes only five units a day over the same time period to potentially start developing symptoms. You are very unlikely to be aware of this though as generally, damage to the liver doesn't show any outward signs.

Take a break and the liver starts to repair and reverse this damage. It's so good at this that according to Danish research even just having one regular alcohol-free day a week allows enough regeneration to reduce risk of cirrhosis[19]. The NHS is a little more conservative and suggests two or three days off to let repair take place. So you might be wondering if the liver can repair a bit in one, two or three days – what happens if you take a month off? The answer according to studies is that the average drinker will reduce the build-up of fat in the liver by 15–20 per cent and liver stiffness – which indicates possible scarring in the liver – could fall by 12.5 per cent.

Your risk of disease falls

Blood pressure also falls when you start drinking. And it doesn't take a month to get this boost – you'll likely see a result in as few as five days. A study of weekend drinkers in Ireland found that after a heavy weekend blood pressure spiked on a Monday but declined throughout the week reaching a low on the Friday[20]. Don't drink again that month and it'll stay low or even fall further.

Abstinence could also lower your risk of developing Type 2 diabetes – a condition reaching epidemic proportions in most Westernised countries. The first stage in the development of

Type 2 diabetes is high levels of glucose (a type of sugar) in the blood and one common cause of this is that our bodies stop responding to the hormone insulin that normally lowers levels of this. However, after a month off alcohol, the *New Scientist* team found their blood glucose levels fell by 16 per cent while the people in the Royal Free trial found their ability to respond to insulin improved by 28 per cent.

Blood cholesterol also falls during a month off and that's a good step toward improved heart health.

As with the benefits to your liver you might not sense any of these changes, but they are happening and your body will thank you for them.

Quitting and Your Weight

Let's move now to something you will be able to see if it occurs – weight loss. On average people lose about 7lb (3kg) abstaining for a month. You can probably work out why without too much prompting: alcohol contains calories – seven calories per gram if you want to be specific – stop drinking and you eliminate these calories and this alone can see you start to lose weight.

How much will depend on what you normally drink. On average, a single measure of spirits with a diet mixer is the lowest calorie tipple at around 60 calories a glass, the most calories are found in cocktails that mix 4–5 shots of spirits alongside sugary or creamy mixers; these can contain over 200 calories a glass. But don't get complacent if your drinks don't come with pun-filled names and umbrellas in the top, two large glasses of wine can contain 370 calories – almost a fifth of the 2,000 calories a woman should have a day.

But as well as the calories in the alcohol to consider, there's also the extra calories in the things you consume as a result of alcohol to take into account. It's recently been discovered that when we're drinking the brain is primed to find food odours appealing – possibly to encourage you to eat and slow down how fast alcohol is absorbed into the system[21]. As such even if you don't intend to eat too much when you start your night out, the smell from the local chip shop while you're waiting for your taxi home is going to be extremely enticing if alcohol is in your system.

Alcohol also stimulates appetite by lowering blood sugar and at the same time lowers your ability to control your actions. When alcohol gets into the brain it dials down our ability to make sensible decisions – all of a sudden that kebab you'd never eat sober seems like a really, really good idea.

If you've just had a couple of glasses or have a strong constitution the damage might stop there, but if you're prone to hangovers you can also expect calorie carnage the morning after.

Have you ever noticed that when hangovers strike, all you want to do is curl up in bed with cups of sweet tea and your own body weight in bacon sandwiches? Or that even if you can't face food when you first wake up, you're eating for England by lunchtime. Truth is hangovers don't just make your head hurt, your limbs shake and your mouth feel like the bottom of a birdcage, they also affect your eating habits and they do so because they send your blood sugar plummeting. Normally when we sleep our body gets fuel from stores of the sugar glucose in the liver, however the presence of alcohol prevents this happening. This causes you to wake up with extra low blood sugar which then triggers your body to start craving food fast to replenish your energy.

And you don't tend to reach for a salad at this point – sugary food, stodgy food or fatty foods tend to be the hangover food of choice. There's no definite reason why this is. Some experts say that alcohol depletes levels of essential fatty acids in the body and you translate this need for good fats into the need for any fat, or it could be some kind of call for help from your body, as fat metabolism produces bile in the liver and bile helps you process alcohol. But it's just as likely that it's psychological – most of us associate fried or greasy foods with comfort – something you need when you've got a hangover.

Eliminate alcohol for a month however and you eliminate the calories you normally consume from it and you avoid the calories you find yourself munching because your inhibition is low or you feel a bit rubbish the morning after – the result of which should be weight loss. I say should though because if you replace alcohol with sugary drinks packed with calories effects will be limited. If you really want to shed pounds as a benefit of giving up booze it's a good idea to mostly stick with soda water or diet sodas when you go out.

How many calories are in your favourite drink?

175ml glass of 13 per cent wine – 159 calories
125ml glass of 12 per cent sparkling wine – 89 calories
330ml bottle of 5 per cent beer – 142 calories

Half a pint of 4 per cent lager – 91 calories

Half a pint of 4.5 per cent cider – 108 calories

Single spirit (without mixer) – 61 calories

Bloody Mary – 150 calories

Margarita – 214 calories

Cosmopolitan – 116 calories

Martini – 204 calories

Pina Colada – 245 calories

Daiquiri – 203 calories

(sources: Drinkaware and Weight Loss Resources Food Database)

Quitting and Your Skin

Look in the mirror – or even better take a picture – before you quit and then compare how you look a week or two later and you'll notice a dramatic difference. You could look 5–10 years younger.

The reason is that alcohol noticeably changes the face. As you drink the blood vessels of the body dilate and in the face where the skin is thin you may notice a red flushing around the cheeks and chin and a slight reddening of the eyes. If this is there regularly you might not think it's abnormal but once you quit you'll rapidly notice your skin looks less ruddy and your eyes are brighter.

You could also notice your face looks thinner as the month goes on. This is another side effect of those enlarged blood vessels which leak watery fluid into the surrounding tissues creating a bloated, puffy look – especially first thing in the morning. As you stop drinking this fluid drains away and your face will slim.

Alcohol also dehydrates the skin and a drier skin is more likely to show fine lines and wrinkles. As these plump back up, you'll turn back the clock on how you look, but you might particularly notice a big difference in the lines between your eyebrows; these can fade or even disappear during your month off and in some people it can even look as if they've had Botox!

To understand why requires delving into Traditional Chinese Medicine. This believes that imbalances in areas of the body show up on specific areas of the face – for example, problems with the lungs show up on the cheeks, the chin is associated with the ovaries. The area between the brows relates to the liver meridian and as such any time you overdo the alcohol you could find lines develop here and, if you're a regular drinker, they may stay put. Quit though, and they vanish. I can tell you that when I give up alcohol one of the first things I notice is that the area between my brows is smoother. In Chinese medicine, dark circles under the eyes can also be related to drinking alcohol and show that your kidneys are a little overworked, these too can disappear during your month off.

Quitting, Wealth and Work

Alcohol costs money. Well, unless you live in the Abruzzo region of Italy where in 2016 one local vineyard set up a free wine fountain – but generally, if you're going to consume alcohol you must pay for it. Don't drink and you'll therefore save money – but you might not realise quite how much.

The benefits to your finances

Let's start with the obvious expenditure; according to the charity Macmillan Cancer Support, the average drinker spends just over £65 a month on alcohol, which immediately gets saved if you're not drinking. On top of that though there're the things you buy while you're under the influence – these might be just little things, the kebab, the chips, the taxi home, or we could talk about a 2014 survey that looked at spending under the influence and found that while the average amount spent during a drunken online shopping spree was £142, one in 20 people wake up to a bill of over £500[22].

You can calculate exactly how much you'd save not drinking online with the Dryathlon Alcohol Calculator at dryathlon.org. Use the slider to pick how many pints, glasses of wine or shots of spirits you drink and it'll calculate how much cash – and calories you'll save during the month. Hopefully you'll think the result isn't too bad for simply forgoing a few hangovers.

Clear heads help your career

A survey by an alcohol delivery company once estimated that in the UK we spend 682 days of our lives nursing hangovers – that's nearly two years[23]. Okay, so people who have booze delivered to their homes might be more prone to overdoing it, so let's look at more independent figures. The Institute of Alcohol Studies estimates that every year lost productivity due to alcohol costs companies £1.7 billion, they also cite a study by Norwich Union Healthcare stating that one in 20 people go to work hungover once a week and a second study by YouGov for medical insurers PruHealth that found 22 per cent of employees made a mistake at work because they were hungover[24]. If that sounds like you, it's probably not doing wonders for your career!

In fact, you could even go as far as to say, hangovers make you stupid. According to research from Keele University you experience a 5–10 per cent drop in the performance of your working memory when hungover[25]. Working memory is the ability to hold information in your mind and manipulate it – something you need to do day-in, day-out if you work with numbers, do coding or fix anything technical as part of your job. On top of this they say the risk of errors increases by 30 per cent when you're hungover. Reaction times are also slower, which could matter if you drive for work, operate machinery or even if your boss asks you a tricky question in that morning meeting.

Partly this is because you're exhausted – remember, alcohol stops you progressing effectively through the cycles of sleep and the stage most affected is that involving REM sleep when the brain restores and consolidates things like memory. This therefore has a negative effect on cognitive function including memory and concentration. Dehydration can also affect how quickly you think and low blood sugar can drain energy and thought processes. Finally, the newest research into hangover suggests many of the symptoms are actually caused by your immune system responding to what it sees as an attack on your body by releasing inflammatory chemicals that cause aches, pains, and, experts believe, the symptoms of mental fog associated with hangover.

All of this disappears if you abstain though. Spend a month going into work clear-headed and who knows how much you could get done or who you might impress.

Diagram of a hangover

One reason that researchers say older people get fewer hangovers is nothing to do with any age-related miracle of metabolism, but is simply down to the fact that with age comes wisdom and the realisation that much of the time, that extra glass of wine or beer is not worth the misery of the morning after. One of THE most easily identifiable benefits of quitting alcohol is not having to wake up with that dry mouth, head pounding, 'Oh dear what exactly did I do?' feeling. If you need a little reminder of exactly how bad it feels, here's our top-to-toe guide to what happens during a hangover and why.

Your head: Headaches are one of the most common symptoms of hangovers. They have two main causes – the dehydrating effects of alcohol causing pain or a reaction to a substance called acetaldehyde which is produced as alcohol metabolises in the body.

Your eyes: When you're tired, the muscles in your eyes get tired, but more importantly, alcohol slows the rate at which you blink. The result is sore, red, tired-looking eyes the morning after.

Your cheeks: Are they burning this morning? If you have a vague recollection of dancing on the bar – or worse, welcome to the embarrassing effects of alcohol. Alcohol suppresses inhibitions so we may do things that we wouldn't have done sober.

Your muscles: So you're aching from head to toe. Blame acetaldehyde, which accumulates in the muscles making you ache. Or did you fall? Alcohol also impairs balance.

Your digestion: Alcohol can either stimulate the bowel leading to diarrhoea or dehydrate stools, which can cause constipation. Fluid and gas can also build up in the stomach leading to bloat. High doses also damage the lining of the stomach, which leads to nausea and sometimes stomach pains.

Quitting and Your Emotions

Most of us associate alcohol with feeling good – after all, you're unlikely to drink if it doesn't give you pleasure. One or two glasses of wine improve mood and take the edge off stress and losing this emotional coping mechanism is often what makes quitting for the month tricky for some. But what people often find is that when their wine (or beer) crutch is taken away they actually spend the month reassessing things about their lives and making changes for the better. After all, if you can't numb your bad day with a drink you're more likely to actually spend a bit of time thinking about what caused it and taking steps to fix it – steps you can use long after the month is over.

For some though alcohol isn't always a nice experience – particularly if you go over those one or two drinks in a session – you might say things you don't mean, do things you regret or get into situations you'd have avoided sober. Giving up immediately frees you from experiencing these negatives. Guilt about what you've consumed, worry about what you did last night or even having to actively apologise for something you said or did, all of these are gone if you don't drink for a month. The fact is alcohol changes our behaviour and some of us don't always like who we become. Quitting for a month puts a brake on this. It can give you time to reassess what alcohol does and how you might be better off without it – or at least with less of it.

Let's take sexual activity as a good example of this. A study from New York University found that alcohol causes more people to have one-night stands with people they wouldn't have found attractive sober than smoking cannabis[26]. Why might be explained by a second study carried out by researchers in Switzerland[27]. They found that the concept of 'beer goggles' – where people look infinitely more attractive when we're drunk – is actually a real thing caused by the combination of alcohol lowering sexual inhibition and making us find anyone who smiles at us more attractive than we would have sober. And even just one pint of beer was enough to cause the 'beer goggle' effect.

And then there's a completely modern morning-after phenomenon you might have to deal with – social media regret. One third of people have put something on social media while drunk that they later regretted – whether this was just because it was littered with spelling mistakes, or something far worse[28]. Avoidance of this is the benefit I enjoy most when not drinking. Personally, I'm a happy drunk – after a couple of wines I decide it's a great idea to plan parties, organise social events and talk to people on social media that I would never dream of communicating with in real life. One of the things I like most about being on the wagon is knowing I can open Instagram/Facebook and Twitter the morning after without a vague sense of dread that I've made a fool of myself in front of potentially millions of people.

The Long-Term Effects

There are many, many more benefits that quitting can have on your body, mind and lifestyle, but if I haven't convinced you of enough benefits by now going on for another 10 pages isn't going to do it, but I will just mention one final thing. Critics of abstinence challenges say they're a bad idea as once they are over people think they can go back to drinking like the proverbial fishes with a clear conscience. The experts say instead, we should be encouraging sensible drinking behaviour year round. Now that is a very good idea, but here's the thing – researchers at the University of

Sussex and Alcohol Concern looked into this[29]. They talked to people six months after they had successfully completed a month off alcohol and found the majority were drinking less and were less likely to 'get drunk' when they did drink.

The fact is, taking a month off drinking helps you break the habit of ordering alcohol on autopilot and teaches strategies that mean even long after your month off is over you're still likely to drink less. Even people who 'slipped up' during the month said taking even some time off helped them make positive changes to their drinking behaviour. Taking a month off works.

So now that you know why you should quit, you want to know how to make it stick. Well, that's where our next chapter comes in. It contains 50 tips that can help you stick at your mission. These come from research studies into quitting drinking and other bad habits or are practically tested tips that have worked for me or friends who've taken time off alcohol. And some of them will work for you too.

CHAPTER TWO

50 Tips to Make Your Month Easy

Deciding to give up alcohol is one thing – actually achieving it can be another as firstly, we fall into habits with drinking – habit is just another word for routine or, if you want to think about it in a slightly more negative way, a rut. We get home from work, we open the fridge, we pour a beer, a glass of wine, a G&T, or whatever your drink of choice might be and we sit down. The working day is done. Ditto, you walk into a pub and, instead of perusing the choices on offer and seeing what you fancy as you would in a restaurant, you just order your usual. Often therefore we're not even truly aware of how much we drink.

The second trigger that causes us to drink is cravings. When we have a drink or two the brain is positively stimulated in areas associated with happiness and reward. After a while we start to connect the two – and for many of us seeing, smelling or even thinking about alcohol (or a place that sells it) causes the urge for a drink. Whether or not you give in to that temptation relies on willpower – and how strong yours is.

Both of these elements will affect how easy giving up alcohol for a month is for you. If you don't have habits associated with alcohol you'll find it far easier than someone who has got into a nightly routine of having a drink. Ditto, if you don't really associate alcohol with pleasure or reward you won't be fighting strong cravings or urges to drink it that require a lot of willpower for you to abstain. In either of these cases, it's very likely that all you'll need to do to successfully quit for a month is use a few of the 50 tips below when you enter a situation in which you would normally drink. These have one aim – to help you make a non-alcoholic choice rather than an alcoholic one. Use one, use two, use all fifty, whatever works best for you ... but do use them.

1. Ask for your soft drink to be served in a wine glass – or a pint glass if you're normally a beer drinker. This is the thing that works every time for me – it tends to stop people asking why you're not drinking (they just see the glass and assume that you are) plus there's something about holding the stem of a wine glass that's satisfying.

2. Ask yourself the big question. If you had the choice to a) go out and drink alcohol but not actually speak to anyone else while you have your drink – or b) go to the pub and see your friends but not drink which would you choose? Most of us choose option b – and if that's the case, you're actually getting the reward from the night out that you want. Remember this when you walk into the pub – you're there to meet your friends, not sink a skin-full.

3. Find a soft drink you like: I soon realised the reason I defaulted immediately to alcohol when I entered a pub is that I don't like the obvious soft drinks on offer – cola, diet cola or fruit drinks are all too sugary for me, so I got creative – most bars have cranberry to mix with vodka and that works just as well with soda – if you're lucky you'll also find elderflower cordial which does a passable impression of white wine when mixed with soda. You'll find 20 more suggestions you can buy in most pubs, or order online if you prefer to 'drink' at home in the box below.

20 Easy Alternatives

If you're not a fan of normal sodas here're 20 more ideas to drink at home or in the pub that can be whipped up, or purchased, without too much effort. You'll also find a list of more complicated Mocktail-like concoctions in the Recipe section starting on page 154.

1. No-alcohol beers like Becks Blue, Bavaria Wit 0.0%, Holsten 0.0%, Carlsberg 0.0% and Ambar 0.0. A beer called St Peters Without comes in a larger 500ml bottle for those who like a pint – and you might even find it on tap in some pubs.
2. You can also make non-alcoholic beers into a shandy with lemonade.

3. Alcohol free ciders. Both Kopperberg and Magners have these in their ranges.

4. Schloer. This sparkling grape juice can substitute for sparkling wine at a push.

5. Tonic water. Gin drinkers this one's for you. You don't actually miss the gin.

6. Red grape juice. It's like sweet red wine.

7. Orange juice and tonic or bitter lemon. The bitterness of the mixers counteracts the sweetness in the juice.

8. Eisberg Alcohol Free Wine. In my opinion, it's the nicest-tasting alcohol-free wine. It works best if it's very, very cold. Add ice.

9. Grapefruit juice and soda.

10. Monin Gin-Flavoured Syrup. It tastes just like the real thing. Try it with soda or tonic.

11. Zeo. This drink was designed to create the same tingle on the tongue as alcohol does. You do find it in some pubs.

12. Chilled herbal tea with lots of ice.

13. Ikea sell an alcohol-free mulled wine.

14. Pink lemonade – lemonade with a splash of grenadine or raspberry syrup.

15. Shirley Temple – ginger beer with a splash of grenadine or raspberry syrup.

16. Bitter lemon – with a salt rim. Wet the glass, dip it in salt, then pour in the bitter lemon – it's kind of like a margarita when you sip it.

17. Kombucha is a super-healthy fermented drink that tastes a bit like wine.

18. Pomegranate and soda. Bars often carry pomegranate juice or syrup for cocktails, just ask them to mix it with soda.

19. Seedlip Non-Alcoholic Spirits. The first range of non-alcoholic drinks designed to suit a spirit drinker's palate; you can order them at seedlipdrinks.com. The site also offers a list of bars that stock them.

20. Shatler's Virgin Cocktail range. Alcohol-free versions of cocktails like Mojitos, Mai Tai and Pina Colada – you'll find these and many other alcohol-free options at alcoholfree.co.uk.

4. If in doubt bring your own – the worst events for me were work lunches or dinners where the only non-alcoholic drink choice was still or sparkling water. That's fine for one or two, but seriously tested my willpower over three to four hours, so I started travelling with a travel-sized bottle (the same as you buy to take shampoo on holiday) filled with elderflower cordial in my handbag and adding that to my water. Squeezy lemon juice that you normally buy to put on pancakes also livens things up brilliantly and is nicely portable.

5. Check out the hashtag HelloSundayMorning on Instagram. It's full of people who have given up booze (for a variety of reasons) sharing what they're doing now they're not hungover. It gives you that extra bit of motivation – and you can post while you join in.

6. Brunch and breakfast are your friend – they're the perfect time to see friends, but don't come loaded with the expectation to drink.

7. Go to a 'dry bar' – there're a few around the country. Some have stand-alone premises, others organise events at different venues around town. At the time of writing some that you might want to check out include

   - Redemption. Have branches in London's Notting Hill and super-trendy Shoreditch (redemptionbar. co.uk)
   - The Brink in Liverpool (thebrinkliverpool.com)
   - The Dry Umbrella in Manchester (facebook.com/ thedryumbrella)
   - Sobar in Nottingham (doubleimpact.org.uk/café-sobar)

8. Avoid rounds – remember, one of the benefits of quitting is that you get to save money that you would have been spending on alcohol, so don't blow cash buying other people booze! But boosting your budget isn't the only reason for avoiding rounds – there's always that one friend who decides you really did want a G&T rather than just a tonic and next thing you know, you're off the wagon.

9. Tap. The tapping technique sees you tapping parts of your body five to seven times. The theory behind it is that many people drink to hide emotions, for example if you're a fairly shy person you'll drink at a party to boost your confidence or, if you're stressed out or unhappy you might have a drink to take the edge off problems you don't want to actually deal with. The idea

of tapping is that you release the energy associated with these emotions and the urge to have a drink goes with them. It might sound a bit far-fetched, but researchers at Mount Sinai St Luke's Hospital in New York tested the technique to fight food cravings and found it helped so it's likely it will work for alcohol cravings too[30]. There are lots of different techniques but the easiest to remember (and do in a pub or bar) is to tap under your eye, then your collarbones while repeating the phrase 'I might want a drink but I don't need one'. Do it five to ten times and feel the cravings disappear.

10. Breathe. Wavering in the off-licence or at a friend's birthday party? Before you make any decision, take two deep breaths and tell yourself to make the right choice for you. At one point during each of my months' off I've thought 'Oh, I've done ten days now, one drink won't hurt'. Taking the deep breaths gave me time to realise that as my aim was to totally quit alcohol for a whole month, one drink would stop that happening.

11. Try mortification. When a craving strikes make a mental list of all the negative experiences you've had while drinking and visualise them in vivid detail. The idea is that you feel so guilty, embarrassed or just ashamed, you realise it would be a very bad idea to drink.

12. Simply keep telling yourself that you don't drink. If you're trying to cut back on anything saying 'No thanks, I don't want it' makes it twice as likely that you'll successfully resist temptation than saying 'No thanks, I can't have that,' finds a study at the US's University of Houston[31]. Saying 'I can't' signals that you're giving up

something desirable but saying 'I don't want it' gives you a sense of empowerment.

13. Offer to drive – everyone loves you so no one nags.

14. Pick pubs with activities – if your mind is distracted by answering questions at the trivia night, playing pool or darts or watching a comedy show you're less likely to feel the call of the bar.

15. Get sponsored. The official month-long abstinence campaigns like Dry January or Ocsober are organised by charities to raise money so not only are you supporting them if you raise money during your month off, you'll also increase your chance of avoiding temptation as you won't want to let your sponsors down.

16. Pledge money to a cause you hate. If you don't want to ask other people to fork out for your success, put your own money where your mouth is – but don't pledge to give it to a cause you believe in, pledge to a cause you don't – a political party you actively dislike for example. You'll be less likely to quit if your failure benefits something negative than if the money is going to a good cause.

17. Make it into a competition: Get the whole office involved and see how many of you can get to the end of the month without drinking – you could even have a plan that the ones that quit have to buy the others lunch or a cake when the challenge is over. In a study by Warwick Business School, competition was shown to help people stick to healthier steps like moving more and eating less – and it's likely to work with avoiding alcohol too.

18. Take an 'alcohol-free' walk home. Research shows that people who live within a kilometer of a pub are 13 per

cent more likely to drink to excess than those who have to travel further to get alcohol[32]. Simply seeing that pub on your way home can trigger cravings that stretch your willpower – so try and find a way home that doesn't pass your local.

19. Book early morning fitness classes or splash some of the cash you're saving on a personal trainer and schedule your sessions for 7am. The idea of trying to exercise that early in the morning feeling a bit jaded should put you off giving in.

20. Create a cash jar. I've talked about how much money you'll save by not drinking so put that cash where your eyes can see it. Get a jar, mark it 'My Sober Fund' and, every night you might have drunk but didn't, put the cash you estimate you might have spent in the jar – and watch it mount up. You can even start making lists of things you want to spend it on when the month is over. If you don't like the idea of a jar full of cash in your home, it works just as well with pebbles – each one representing a pound. You'll still see the amount in the jar mount up.

21. Clear the alcohol out of your house before you start – or at least put it somewhere you can't see it. In the same way that walking past the pub triggers booze cravings, so does seeing a bottle of wine in the fridge. Again, proof that this works comes from weight-loss research – people who could see sweets in their office ate twice as many than when the sweets were hidden[33].

22. Fill your evenings. Often we drink out of boredom but if you fill your evenings you won't have time to get bored. Here's a list of some of the things I plan to do during months off – admittedly some of them are

more fun than others, but they all give me a sense of accomplishment.

- Edit your holiday photos. I'm not a great photographer but I'm marvelous on the photo editing software Picassa.
- Do your accounts – I told you some of these things weren't that much fun.
- Clear out your clutter – I firmly recommend the book *The Life-Changing Magic of Tidying* by Marie Kondo (Vermilion) for this task. It changes the whole way you think about decluttering.
- Arrange your bookshelf by colour – it's strangely satisfying and looks really arty.
- Write a book – at least part of this manuscript was completed during evenings of abstinence.
- Plan your holiday – I mean really plan it. I have a list of 20 bars I want to visit, 20 restaurants I want to visit, off-the-beaten track activities to try – I even look up train schedules. I don't necessarily do all these things but I spend hours planning.
- Learn something – a language, a skill, computer code.
- Netflix – get a 30-day subscription and binge-watch EVERYTHING.
- Go the library – don't laugh. I know we have e-readers now, but the library is free and it allows you to pick up books you might not want to take a chance spending money on. My rule is I walk in and pick up the first five books that catch my eye no matter what they're on. If you don't enjoy them you

just take them back a week or two later.

- Start a blog – my posts while not drinking are still among the most popular posts I've written on mine.
- Cook meals from scratch – you'll still have something tasty to look forward to each night.
- Exercise – but aim for a goal – like trying to swim a kilometer in laps.
- Empty your e-reader – talking of reading you know those books you bought two years ago and never got time to read … now is the time.
- Pamper yourself. I often complain I don't have time to paint my toenails until it comes to abstinence month!

23. Set a challenge. How many new places can you go that don't have anything to do with alcohol? Now is the time to experiment. Think cafes, coffee shops, poetry readings in bookshops, bowling, the cinema, museums, the park, the swimming pool, even just go for a walk to fill the time.

24. Change your password. If every time you sign into your email you type 'Nodrinks2day', it's reinforcing in your head the choice you've made. There's an entire movement in the USA called 'positive passwording' looking into the psychology of this tiny tweak and how it can change people's lives.

25. Make a reasons list. Most people don't just quit for the sake of it – make a list of all the reasons behind why you're giving up for a while, you could even set yourself a number like 25, 50 or 100 and try and find enough reasons to fill it. Refer to that if your willpower starts to fade.

26. Do a Benefits Audit. Check in each day and list three benefits you can see about staying on the wagon. Are you waking up and checking your social media free from a sense of dread? Does your skin look better? Have you lost a pound or two? If you focus on the positive changes you're less likely to want to stop them happening by taking a drink.

27. Leave an event before you get bored. If you're bored, you're far more likely to reach for alcohol in order to numb the feeling – or to try and liven things up a bit.

28. Vary your drinks. If you go into a bar and decide to drink soda all night, it can get very boring, very fast. So, mix and match your orders.

29. Don't go to the bar yourself – send a trusted friend to order your virgin drink of choice.

30. Put your goals on social media. And take note of the likes. It helps you achieve your goal says a study from New York University. In the trial they found that people telling others that they were going to achieve something were spurred on when other people took notice of their behaviour[34].

31. Repeat the following mantra: 'It will all still be there in 31 days,' or however many days you have left. Pubs, clubs, bars and the booze aisle at the supermarket are not going anywhere. Once your month is over you can reach for whichever tipple takes you fancy. Of course, if they announce Prohibition while you're taking your month off, then it's fine to give in to your urge.

32. Wait 15 minutes. Most of the time the need to drink is merely a craving. Cravings are funny things, they hit very quickly, they hit hard, they consume your thoughts and they're often weirdly specific. But if you can distract your

mind and stop thinking about them they will also pass – normally within 15 minutes. You'll find some more advice on busting cravings in Chapter Four.

33. Pay for some evening activities. Buy theatre or cinema tickets, book a weekly spin class or language lessons all in advance – if you're already spent the cash you won't be tempted to skip what you had planned to go down the pub instead.

34. Get supporters to send you text messages. Smokers trying to quit were more likely to succeed when researchers sent them motivating texts[35]. The same thing has been shown for people starting exercise regimes. If you have other friends also giving up for the month send each other tips and tricks that you find are working for you.

35. Tighten a muscle. If you're starting to waver, simply clench your bicep, tighten your calves or clench your buttocks – research published in the *Journal of Consumer Research* found that tightening muscles actually increases resilience and willpower[36].

36. Do a Power Pose. If you start to feel your willpower waning, go to the bathroom and stand with your arms up over your head in a victory pose. It's claimed this helps send blood to the brain that allows you to think more clearly – plus, you'll have removed yourself from the situation, which is another good way of stopping yourself doing something you'll regret later.

37. Don't go the pub grumpy. You're less likely to make healthy choices if you're in a bad mood. A bad mood causes us to forget the wider picture and focus only what's right in front of us – i.e. how a drink will make us

feel right now. If you can't change your mood completely, at least think of something happy before you place your order. This has been shown to help people eat less – and is also likely to help change habits in other ways.

38. Choose your buddies carefully. Are they likely to nurse one glass of wine all night, or more likely to down a bottle and sulk if you're not drinking with them. The latter are far more likely to try and coerce you to booze. It's been clearly shown that we tend to mimic the behaviour of people we're with – so try and stick with good influences for this month.

39. Shut down Tinder. When we're out with people that we are trying to impress, like a first date or your boss, we're more likely to consume things that we don't actually want, due to our need to seek approval. It's a good idea to stick to people who you can be yourself around while trying to quit.

40. Go to brightly lit places. Or sit by the window. You make healthier choices in brightly lit environments as light raises self control say US researchers.

41. Avoid any activity you *need* drink to take part in. I learnt this little trick back in the 1990s when I had a boyfriend who loved raves. I hated them. I would therefore have more drinks than I needed to get through the night. For the next month say no to things that you think you'd need a drink to get through – depending on your personality this might include dinner parties, work events where you don't know anyone, house parties or karaoke.

42. Shake your head. Actually shaking your head no as you make the decision to turn something down helps reinforce your decision found researchers at the US's Ohio University and Spain's Autonomous University of Madrid[37].

43. Eat something. One common reason you crave alcohol is that your blood sugar is low and your brain translates this into a craving for sugar or alcohol (which is basically sugar in liquid form). If a craving is happening, try eating a snack of something tasty and filling like cheese and biscuits, Greek yogurt and berries or houmous and crudités. It will distract you from the thought of alcohol and also raise your blood sugar.

44. Visualise. Imagine walking into a pub or coming home at night and ordering/pouring a soft drink. And when I say imagine, I really mean imagine – look around you and see the room in intricate detail – the colour of the walls, the furniture, even who else is there. Feel your feet on the carpet walking to the bar. Hear the sounds around you as you open the bottle of drink or the words you say to order it. Now imagine feeling the cold glass in your hand, taste how refreshing that first mouthful is and how good you feel that you have a soft drink in your hand instead of an alcoholic one. If you do all of that you're more likely to succeed than someone who just decides that's what they're going to do and doesn't use visualisation say researchers at Canada's McGill University[38].

45. Order first when out in a group. You're more likely to stick to the choice you actually want to make if you do. One very good trick if you're out for dinner is to arrive five minutes before everyone else and order at least one big bottle of sparkling water for the table. Then get the waiter to take your wine glass away.

46. Don't apologise for being boring: that just reinforces in your mind that what you're doing is a negative thing.

Look forward to whatever you're doing that night and relish the fact that you don't need alcohol to enjoy it.

47. Remember you're not alone. If you're doing one of the organised months like Dry January or Ocsober chances are you aren't the only person in the venue not drinking. Nor does the bar staff care if you're ordering soda water – they're probably happy to realise they have one less person to keep an eye on/order a taxi for/find their shoes at 3am.

48. Ask this question before you cheat: 'How will this make me feel an hour after I drink it?' If the answer is guilty, grumpy, defeated and like you've failed, then don't drink it.

49. Go to a completely different pub from your usual haunt: Habits are triggered by routine – psychologists say the best time to break a habit is when you move house or change job as you won't fall into the same traps you always do. For this reason, it's going to be easier to order a soft drink somewhere you're not used to visiting than in your local.

50. Just aim to get through today. If a month without alcohol seems insurmountable, don't think about it that way. Goals are often easier if we break them down into small chunks – the more immediate and achievable the goal, the more likely you are to achieve it. Setting the goal when you wake up in the morning to just not drink that day might work better for you than telling yourself you're not going to drink for a month.

Hopefully, all of that should arm you with enough tactics to beat temptation, but if you do slip up – there's one final thing to remember. Give up the idea of all or nothing: If you do slip off the wagon, then don't think of it as a failure. If you have one night where you drink, that's not a big deal if you still manage to stay off the sauce for the other 30 days, so just start again. I admit to doing this while writing this book. I'd done eleven and three-quarter days without drinking and I was out socialising for almost all of them – I currently live in Australia where I haven't yet found a pub that sells non-alcoholic beer and this night I'd had four lime and sodas and I just wanted to drink something that wasn't sweet and so I had a light beer. It was a conscious decision and actually I didn't enjoy it much. I therefore got straight back on track the next day – and that was what mattered. Yes I'd had one drink, but I still had 19 more days of saying no ahead of me. I referred to it in my obligatory Facebook confession as doing 'Damp January'.

For some people using a selection of the tips in this chapter will be all you need to get you to the end of the month without touching a drop, others however might need a little bit more help. The more habitual your drinking, the harder saying no is going to be to do as you've got to consciously change a behaviour that's quite firmly entrenched in your routine – and you might not even really understand why. But don't worry, experts love to investigate the science of habits and how to break them, so there's plenty of advice out there to turn to. The next chapter explores it.

CHAPTER THREE

Habits – and How to Break Them

When researchers at the University of Sussex investigated what types of people were most successful at abstaining from alcohol for the whole month of a challenge they found it was those who drank only moderately or irregularly before the challenge began[39]. One reason for this is that it's likely they were still at the stage where drinking alcohol was a conscious choice and not a habit and it's a lot easier to change a behaviour you're consciously aware of than one done partly on autopilot.

Every day we do things that are habitual: brushing your teeth, getting off the bus at a certain stop, buying the same brand of yogurt you always do without even considering the other 20 on the shelf. You weren't born doing all of these things, you learnt to do them, repeating them until they became a normal part of your daily routine – and that's what a habit is, a behaviour repeated regularly and often uncon-sciously. It's been estimated that 40 per cent of the things we do each day are habitual rather than conscious choices[40].

Developing habits is actually our brain trying to protect itself. Every second of every day our brain is juggling input from the thousands of sights, sounds and smells around us. On top of that, it's focusing on keeping us alive, upright, and moving while making decisions and carrying out actions. If we paid close attention to every single one of the thoughts, feelings, sounds, sights, etc. generated while doing all this, we'd never get anything done – even the simple act of getting on the bus or buying that yogurt would overwhelm us. As such, our brain develops a kind of filter system. It ignores some thoughts entirely, it develops the ability to action repetitive tasks without consciously think-ing about them, and once you start to repeat something over and over again your brain stops it being a conscious choice and eventually turns it into an entrenched behav-iour that you then do on autopilot. When this is a positive thing like brushing your teeth or going for a run, this isn't a problem – but if it's one of those things we tend to think about more negatively, like smoking, eating sugary snacks, biting our nails, or drinking more often than we should, it becomes more of a problem.

How habits develop

Habits form in three stages. Stage one is exploring a new behaviour – you try something, the brain examines it and decides if it likes it or not. If you never do this thing again the brain forgets about it, but if you repeat a behaviour, particularly one the brain likes, neurological pathways develop in the brain that, over time, help turn a conscious choice into something we see as routine. As it does this, to save its thought processes further, the brain clumps actions repeated in series together – so, say for example you come home from work, kick off your shoes, walk to get a glass of wine and sit down. If you do that night after night after night eventually your brain clumps these steps together as one task – in time, you don't even think about whether you actually want your glass of wine that evening. Once you kick off your shoes, you simply reach into the fridge and grab it. Now you've got a habit.

Anything can become a habit, but alcohol triggers some specific effects in the brain that make drinking it a particularly easy habit to form. Habits become more ingrained if we are rewarded by them in some way, and alcohol offers us plenty of rewards starting with the fact that it's made from sugar – and sweet things create positive sensations in the brain that give us pleasure. Alcohol also triggers the release of the neurotransmitter dopamine in the reward centre of your brain. Dopamine has been described as the chemical of sin – it's the chemical released when you take drugs, have sex and during orgasm. It makes us feel good. The more you start to release dopamine, the more you crave its effects, and the substances or experiences that provide it.

Alcohol also causes us to release endorphins, another set of neurochemicals that makes us feel good, and the more you drink, the more endorphins you produce. In addition, heavy drinking causes damage to the connections between the parts of the brain that control self-regulation and impulse control. As such, the more you drink the harder stopping might feel. But just because something is hard, it doesn't mean it's impossible. Every habit is breakable – if you know how.

Breaking habits – the brain-friendly guide

Scientists now have the ability to look into the brain as it works without harming it. This allows them to see exactly which parts of the brain light up during a particular thought – and what's been discovered about habits recently is interesting. While at a conscious thought level we don't register when we're about to do something habitual, subconsciously the brain *does* register what we're doing and a part of the brain called the neocortex lights up. If you stimulate that part of the brain, you can stop a habit in its tracks and very quickly break it. What this shows is that even the most ingrained habit has an on-off switch that's ready to be triggered if we just take a second to think about what we're doing before we do it. Bringing a habit into your consciousness is the first step in being able to break it. The good news is that the very act of picking up this book and making the decision to quit for a month alerts your conscious that you're hoping to make a change. Now it's time to act on that.

Scientists refer to the brain as having plasticity – it's constantly changing, growing and forming new connections – and when you start to regularly make a different choice in a situation rewiring begins. Say now you walk in through the door, kick off your shoes and go and have a hot shower before you sit down and relax instead of reaching for your normal nightly drink. The reward of feeling good from the shower means your brain thinks this is a behaviour it might like to encourage and so it starts to create a new feedback loop. The more you repeat the behaviour the stronger this loop becomes and, eventually, you create a new habit. Think of it like walking through a field – you start off taking the well-worn path never disturbing the fresh grass either side of you. Then, one day a hole opens up in the middle of that path so you have to deviate onto the fresh grass to get to where you're going. The first time you walk that way, the grass springs back up as if you've never been there – but after a week of treading that new path over and over, the grass is flat and you can clearly see where you're going. Eventually, the old path starts to grow new grass and you can't see that as clearly any more – but no matter, as the new path is now second nature to walk down. That's exactly what happens in the brain when you change a habit. The more you repeat the behaviour, the more it becomes your new normal.

Before we investigate further how to create this new path (and your new normal) though, there's a myth to dispel. You often hear that habits take 28 days to break. Not necessarily. A study at University College London asked people to make a selection of different changes involving eating, drinking or doing a new activity and measured exactly how long it took before the behaviour become automatic, and the answer was anything from 18 to 254 days with 66 days being the average[41]. As such, some people might need more than one month to completely break the habit of drinking but your time off will give you a very good head start.

The Steps That Break a Habit

It takes three stages to form a habit but there're four parts involved in breaking one.

1. You have something that triggers the habitual behaviour
2. You have a routine that makes it happen
3. You get a reward from carrying it out
4. You need to be satisfied with your choice.

So, with drinking, for example, the trigger might be having a stressful day at work, and the routine is you then ring your friend who is always up for a beer and arrange to meet them in the pub, the reward is that a pint takes the edge off your jangly nerves – and you get to rant about your day with someone who will listen. Breaking a habit can involve intervening at any (or all) of these points.

Step one: Finding your trigger

Habitual behaviours are often triggered by something – it might be a place, a time, a person or an activity that you start to associate with alcohol. For example, if you always have a drink while watching *Strictly Come Dancing* on a Saturday night, eventually when you switch on and simply hear the theme music, you'll start fancying a drink – watching the show without a glass in your hand won't feel quite right. Spotting what triggers you to drink and changing it is the first step in breaking the habit.

For some people the trigger is obvious – you always drink when you've had a bad day, in front of the television or with a certain friend. These triggers are easy to spot and therefore easy to try and change. Sometimes though, triggers aren't quite so easy to spot, there's no obvious immediate cause and effect that means you habitually choose to drink.

This was me during my first ever month of quitting. I'd been paid by a magazine to write an article on how to stop drinking, but still keep up my social life. That meant hibernating was not an option and I had to go out and socialise. The first time I walked into a bar teetotal I had absolutely no idea what I wanted to order. I don't like sugary drinks nor did I want to consume the calories they contained, the diet drink selection in this bar was limited and I was absolutely stuck. I realised I didn't drink alcohol in a pub because I desperately wanted it, but because I couldn't think of an alternative I liked. If I was going to consume calories, I'd prefer them in the form of wine or lager than a sugary cola. It was a life-changing moment and one that has been key to my successful quitting missions ever since as I now have a list of possible no-alcohol alternatives stashed in my brain to call on when required (see 20 Easy Alternatives on page 31).

So, what do you think triggers you to drink? Try and make a list of as many things as possible and then think about ways you can change your behaviour to avoid each trigger. If you're stuck, then spend a few weeks keeping a 'Why Do I Do It' diary. What you're going to need to note down is the following information every time you have – or crave – a drink.

- What time/day is it?
- What mood are you in?
- Where are you?

- Who are you with?
- What are you doing at that time?
- What did you do just before it?
- Why do you think you want a drink?

As you examine this you'll soon spot patterns that trigger your habit – and you can start to alter your behaviour to avoid that trigger. So, using our *Strictly* example above, if you realise you've got into a habit of drinking in front of a particular TV show, you could think about watching it on 'catch-up TV' the next morning when you're less likely to feel like a drink. You could make sure that you simply don't have booze in the house on a Saturday night. You could try sitting on a different chair from the one you normally use – even a change that small can break a habit. Once you find your trigger, focus on finding a way to eliminate it and you'll be a step closer to breaking your habit.

Ideally, for optimum success you'll complete your 'Why Do I Do It' diary and analyse your behaviour to find your trigger for a few weeks before your month off, but if it's too late for that and you're reading this on day one of your month-off mission, that's okay, you can also fill it in as cravings strike and learn as you go.

Step two: Change your routine

Alcohol does not come out of the tap – if you don't go to the pub, the off-licence or the supermarket, you won't be able to get any. Not buying booze and staying away from places that sell it is therefore the simplest way to change the routine that sees you drinking. Some people actually enjoy the rest staying at home gives them, but what if you *do* want to go out and socialise during your month off? Then you need to break your routine in other ways and there're a few different approaches proven to help here. It's just a matter of finding which one, or combination, works best for you …

The Approach: If–Then

The If–Then approach allows you to come up with alternative behaviours when the urge to drink strikes. All you have to do is think of some situations in which you might normally fall into the routine of having a drink – and come up with a plan of action of how you are going to act if the situation arises using the phrase If–Then. So, for example, you might say …

If … the people at work invite me to the pub at lunchtime
Then … I will say I'm meeting a friend already

If … I get home from work stressed out
Then … I will run a bath and use that bath oil I save for special occasions.

If … My friend moans that I'm not drinking
Then … I will lie and say I've got to drive at 6am tomorrow morning.

For this approach to work however you need to make sure of a couple of things: the activity you are going to perform if something happens has to be doable – there's no point promising yourself a bath if you don't have one. On top of this, you're more likely to have success with the If–Then approach if the second half of your statement is positive. So instead of saying 'If the people from work invite me to the pub at lunchtime then I will tell them I can't come', come up with a solution along the lines of 'If the people from work invite me to the pub at lunchtime, then I will say "Not this time," and go that little cafe I love for lunch instead.' Don't focus on what you can't do; think about what you can, particularly if it will give you pleasure.

The Approach: Pause Button Therapy®

The approach of Pause Button Therapy®, or PBT as it's also known, was created by therapists Martin and Marion Shirran to help their clients break the habit of overeating. But they soon discovered it could play a role in helping people break all sorts of habits. The technique is explained fully in their book *Pause Button Therapy*®[42] but I'll describe it briefly here. The next time you're thinking about making a choice that could negatively impact on achieving your goal, conjure up the image of a remote control in your head. Now mentally press the buttons to do the following:

Push Pause – see yourself exactly as you are but imagine time has stood still.

Now, mentally Fast Forward into the future – be it an hour or a day and see, smell and feel the results of the choice you currently think you're about to make.

Rewind back to the present and then, Fast Forward again using a different choice – is it a better outcome?

Rewind to the present and using that knowledge determine the action to take.

Press Play and get on with your life – ideally without a drink in your hand.

The Approach: Aversion Therapy

Did you bite your nails when you were little? If so, there's a good chance that at some point your parents tried painting them with something nasty tasting so that every time you put your fingers in your mouth to chomp it tasted horrible. If that sounds familiar then, congratulations you've already been exposed to the concept of aversion therapy – and if you still don't bite your nails you'll see it can work.

The principle is simple – if you start to associate a habit with something unpleasant, your brain no longer feels rewarded and you'll be less likely to want to do it. You might even start to actively dislike whatever you're trying to avoid as happened to a group of drinkers given electric shocks in one trial. Afterwards they found even the idea of alcohol repugnant[43].

The good news is you don't need to resort to electric shocks to get results, you can simply place a rubber band around your wrist and whenever you develop the urge to drink then ping the band telling yourself to 'STOP'. You'll soon start to associate the thought of alcohol with an unpleasant sensation, which can help stop cravings. The pinging sensation is also very good at bringing the thought of drinking into your conscious mind – which then allows you to use a tactic like Pause Button Therapy® to help you reassess the choice you're about to make.

The Approach: Find Your New Path

One mistake people commonly make when they try and break a habit is just to stop trying to do it. This doesn't work. Remember, a habit is a well-worn path in your brain and to counteract it you need to come up with a new pathway for your thoughts to walk down and you do this by finding alternatives to elements of the habit you're going to break.

In the case of not drinking, exactly what these alternatives need to be depends on how you're going to handle your month off.

Are you still going to go to the pub, parties or out for dinner? If you are, then your new pathway involves finding a new choice of drink to order when you go out. So spend the next five minutes making a list of as many as you can think of that you might enjoy – check the list in Chapter Two (see page 31) if you need some ideas. Take your list out with you and actively consult it before you order. In a study carried out by researchers in the US and Spain[44], people actually carrying the list of benefits of a plan they had decided to follow were more likely to successfully make choices based upon the plan than those who'd just read about the benefits of following it.

Are you going to avoid the pub? Then, your alternatives are likely to be related to what activities you can do instead. These might be things you can do with friends that don't involve any alcohol – or ways to pass your time in the evening at home that you don't associate with sitting down with a drink. Again, the key is to make the biggest list you can think of so that when temptation strikes, you have alternatives in place.

Are you simply going to avoid bad influences? If so, who are you going to spend time with this month instead? And how are you going to handle any invites from those that it might not be healthy to spend time with? This is a good time to start using the If-Then approach so you know exactly how to respond when situations occur.

Step three: Replace the reward you get from alcohol

We drink alcohol because we get something from it. That reward might come from the pleasant sensations associated with alcohol itself, or the circumstances in which we drink it. For example: my partner and I both work from home. My office is upstairs, his is downstairs. About 4.30pm most evenings I get an instant message from him saying 'Pub?' On the face of it you might think my partner is a tiny bit addicted to alcohol – but that isn't the case. What he (and I, because most of the time I give in) actually want from our outing is not alcohol but the reward of leaving the house, of seeing a view that isn't our own four walls – and, if we're very lucky, speaking to someone other than just each other, and where we used to live going to the pub was a cheap, easy way of achieving this. Thankfully we now live a 20-minute walk away from an amazing Asian Food Court so at the beginning of the week at least now the message often reads 'Laksa?' or 'Pho?' instead. Identifying exactly what you're getting from alcohol and replacing that with something else can therefore make quitting much easier. The 'Why Do I Do It' diary in step one can help you find your reward as well as your trigger.

Once you determine what your reward is, then make a list of as many things that could create that sensation instead and start to turn to them when you'd normally try and tackle a feeling with alcohol. Carry that list with you and refer to it whenever you feel you need to reward yourself with alcohol. Yes, I'm aware that by this point you might be carrying around a lot of pieces of paper.

Step four: Be satisfied with your choice

When you're attempting to make any change in life, knowing what the benefits are for you is fundamental in making that change long term. The way to measure this when you're quitting alcohol is to come up with a list of all the benefits you're getting from not consuming it. I've already suggested this as a quick tip in the last chapter so you might already have tried it, but if it's not speaking to you then it's time to tweak the approach slightly.

Psychologists say that the world of change is divided into two types of people: those who are motivated by preventing the negative effects of a bad habit – which they refer to as 'prevention focused', and those who are motivated by the positive benefits that come from stopping that habit – which they refer to as 'promotion focused'. People with strong habits get better results when their list of benefits is worded in the way that taps into their personal motivational type[45].

To try and work out which you are look at the pairs of statements and see which appeals the most – statement A or statement B.

1. a) I want to quit alcohol as it will stop me ageing as quickly
   b) I want to quit alcohol as it will make my skin look younger
2. a) I want to quit alcohol as it will stop me feeling hungover
   b) I want to quit alcohol as it will help me perform better at work
3. a) I want to quit alcohol as it will stop me gaining weight
   b) I want to quit alcohol as I will lose weight
4. a) I want to quit alcohol as it will stop me overspending
   b) I want to quit alcohol as I will have more money at the end of the week
5. a) I want to quit alcohol as it will reduce damage to my liver
   b) I want to quit alcohol as it will improve health

If you ticked mostly A statements you're more 'prevention focused' and motivated by avoiding the negative effects you might get from alcohol so when making your list of reasons, try to word them to pinpoint all the negatives you might avoid by sticking to your month off. If however, you ticked mostly Bs you are 'promotion focused' and motivated more by promoting the positive benefits of quitting so now, when you think of your benefits list really try and turn them into positive statements focusing on what you'll gain or achieve if you stick with your plan.

When Alcohol Becomes a Problem

Before we move on to the next chapter, there's one extremely important thing I have to mention about the habit of drinking, the fact that alcohol is addictive and it's possible to develop a dependency upon it. If you have an addiction or dependency on alcohol it's *not* recommended that you try the month-off approach. Giving up alcohol suddenly is not suitable for anyone who has a genuine dependency on alcohol as withdrawal can be very tough on the body and potentially even harmful.

Recognising the signs of a dependency

The signs of a dependency include:

- An overriding preoccupation with drinking and where your next drink is coming from.
- Having a compulsive need for a drink – and finding it hard to stop once you start.
- Waking up and drinking – or feeling like you need a drink in the morning.
- The need to drink interferes with other elements of your life like work or relationships.
- You have withdrawal symptoms like shaking,

sweating or nausea which subside if you drink again.

If this sounds like you, then it's important to work with your doctor, a mental health professional or other professional alcohol service when you first try to quit. Organisations like Alcoholics Anonymous can then help you adjust to a life of sobriety long term.

The world of addiction used to be black and white, however there's now a grey area that some psychologists are calling 'almost addiction'. The definition of this is that a person is using alcohol – or another substance – in a way that's negative, but is not yet dependent upon it. They might go days or even weeks without drinking, but when they do, their behaviour isn't healthy. Signs of an 'almost addiction' include feeling guilty or regretful after drinking, consuming more than you know is good for you, not being able to stop when you start, keeping secret or lying to others about how much you drink and knowing you'd feel better physically or emotionally if you'd cut back. For you, trying a month off can be very helpful. It allows you to you break the habits that trigger unconscious drinking behaviour, lets you develop alternatives to alcohol for coping with situations like stress and completely reassess your relationship with alcohol.

You may decide that actually you don't want to go back to drinking when the month is over, that your health, relationships, career or other areas of your life will benefit more from you abstaining most of the time. In this case, organisations like Club Soda (joinclubsoda.co.uk) can help you stay focused. Formed by someone who quit drinking, but didn't feel Alcoholics Anonymous was right for her, it provides support for people who want to stay sober, but don't feel the more intense groups are right for them.

No matter what your relationship with alcohol though, there's an important point I have to keep mentioning. A sober month is not an excuse to drink heavily the other eleven months of the year; it doesn't act as a 'get out of jail free' card for the health of your liver or the rest of your body. The whole point of this month off is to reassess your intake and change your habits so you drink sensibly the rest of the time too.

Right lecture over – let's move on. Now it's time to talk about the gremlin that can throw a spanner into the works of even the best of alcohol-free intentions: temptation and its countermeasure, willpower. I call temptation a gremlin because that's what it feels like – an evil little creature that sits on your shoulder and says 'Go on, have a drink, just one drink'. You then have to conjure up something that kills the gremlin, and that something is willpower. Many of us feel willpower is the most important thing to possess when trying to carry out a challenge like a month of drinking. Actually, scientists say breaking the habits is the most important thing, which is why I've talked about this first, but that doesn't mean willpower doesn't play a role – it's definitely something you'll use and it's definitely something you need to understand.

CHAPTER FOUR

Willpower – and How to Get It

B ack in the 1960s and 70s an interesting set of experiments was carried out in the US. A small child was put in a room and given either a marshmallow or a cookie. They were told if they could wait just 15 minutes without eating the treat in front of them, they could have two treats when the researcher came back.

What happened next varied – some children totally ignored the marshmallow, some covered it up so they couldn't see it, others ate it immediately not caring about the prize to come. A few tried licking the marshmallow figuring that wasn't technically eating it. My favourite result though was the ones that sat there stroking it like it was a stuffed animal. Only a third of over 600 children tested lasted long enough to get the second treat!

The test, of course, determined self-control (aka willpower) and whether people would be willing to forgo instant gratification for a bigger prize later on. Years later the researchers followed up the children and found those with the highest self-control tended to have better exam scores, better social skills, lower weight and be less likely to have problems with drug or alcohol abuse. It seemed that being able to delay the gratification of instant pleasure for the greater reward of reaching a goal has some major benefits in life.

Fast forward over 50 years and scientists are still studying willpower and self-control – and they can still divide children (and adults) into strokers, snatchers and the iron-willed self-controlled. And goals like spending a month without alcohol STILL require the ability to delay instant gratification for the pursuit of a greater long-term gain. But over the years we've learnt more about what's going on in the brain to allow that to happen and how we can alter our willpower levels – and the good news is, we all have enough willpower to meet our goals if we know how to use it.

Willpower examined

Willpower is the energy we use to resist short-term temptations in order to meet a long-term goal – you could also call it self-control or self-discipline. Think of it as like juggling two parts of you – the part that wants pleasure or reward now – and the part that understands that avoiding pleasure for a little while will bring greater benefit in the future. We spend much of our time juggling these two parts – it's just a matter of which one wins in any given situation.

When it comes to sticking to something like a month off alcohol, having good willpower helps – in fact, most of us think it's THE most important element in making successful change[46]. But here's something that might surprise you – particularly if you think you have low levels of willpower. Willpower is not an individualised substance. The willpower you use to get up and go to work each day or brush your teeth before bed when you're really tired draws from exactly the same pool as that which you draw on to say no to chocolate, get yourself to the gym, to say no to booze for a month. Unless you spend each day in a hedonistic wonderland where you do exactly what feels best for you from the minute you get up until you fall asleep to heck with convention and responsibilities, you do have enough willpower to achieve your goal. You've just got to make sure it's allocated correctly.

Work your Willpower Muscle

Imagine an ink pen that automatically refills every night. It starts off full, but every time you use it, the ink level gets depleted and, at some point, it ends up empty. This is exactly like your willpower. You wake up brimming with it, but throughout the day you draw upon it and levels fall and, eventually, levels get so low your brain stops allocating willpower to certain tasks and your resolve starts to waver. How easy you'll find it to resist temptation therefore depends on three things – how much willpower you start with, how much you use throughout your day and if you refill your supply at any point.

Let's start with your base level. We don't all wake up with the same size pen (if you'll allow me to continue using that analogy). The marshmallow test clearly showed that some people are born with a greater propensity for will than others. What determines this base level of willpower is still being teased out. There's a belief there's a genetic element to it but it's possible it's also related to how your brain is wired. In people with strong willpower, decisions are mostly controlled by an area of the brain called the prefrontal cortex, which is involved with complex thinking. In people with low willpower, however, another area of the brain is more dominant – the ventral striatum which is normally involved in fulfilling desire or reward. If that part of the brain is more active you'll be more likely to put short-term pleasure ahead of any delayed gratification from reaching your goal.

But while this set point determines your general range of willpower, exactly how readily you'll give in to temptation when it arises varies day-to-day depends on how often you use your supply and generally, we use it a lot. It's estimated that in an average day we spend three to four hours resisting doing something we want to[47] and every one of these choices drains willpower slightly. These choices might be things like going to work instead of staying in bed, forgoing a biscuit with your morning cup of tea, not telling your boss that you think he's an idiot. But willpower doesn't just get depleted by these 'sensible' decisions, every decision we make taxes it – ponder what shoes you should wear that morning and a bit disappears, stick your head out the door to determine whether you need a coat or not and that's another bit gone, spend a few minutes deciding whether to reply to that email now or wait half an hour until you've got a bit more information and you sapped another part of your reserve – no wonder that by the time you get to the pub at night you find it hard to say no to a drink. Your willpower is in your boots.

While decision fatigue is the main factor that reduces willpower, it's not the *only* thing to affect it. Hunger and how much glucose is in your system also play a role. Glucose is a sugar that you form from food and it's your brain's preferred source of fuel. If your glucose levels are low you'll find it harder to make the best choice – so much so, that numerous studies have shown that when researchers have given people with low willpower a sugary drink during a task they've managed to keep going far longer than they suspected they could[48]. The sugary drink literally refilled their willpower supply. While I'm not suggesting you start turning to sugary drinks to stick to your challenge, it is important during your month off that you try not to skip meals and focus on foods that keep your blood sugars steady (more on that in the diet plan you'll find in Chapter Six).

Uncertainty also seems to sap willpower – if you're not sure about a choice you're about to make, you're more likely to waver on it say researchers at the University of Pennsylvania[49] so, if you haven't written that list of reasons as to why you're quitting alcohol yet, here's another prompt to do it. It'll eliminate any uncertainty that you're making a choice that's not right for you.

Strengthening Your Willpower

The good news is, just as willpower can be depleted by what's happening around us, we can strengthen it too – top up your pen's ink supply if you like.

The most important element in doing this is to limit the decisions you make each day. Mark Zuckerberg, founder of Facebook, is famed for the fact that his daily wardrobe consists of an identical grey t-shirt – but he says not having to decide what to wear each day frees up mental energy for more important decisions. Admittedly for some of us, clothes are fun and wearing the same thing day in, day out, isn't the right solution to keep our headspace clear, but all of us have some decisions we can make each day that we can eliminate. So, ask yourself – what don't I need to have to think about each day and how can I make that happen? For example:

Do you really need to pick between three different cereals each day – or could you just pick one healthy breakfast and eat that every day?

Do you spend ages deliberating over your evening meal each night – or could you cook seven meals on a Sunday, label them by day, eat them as directed?

Do you debate whether you're going to go to the gym every day – or could you write your sessions in your diary each week and just simply stick with them or join a class that meets a set time so any decision on timing is made for you?

Another way to handle relatively unimportant decisions like what to wear to work the next day is to make them shortly before bed, when you're using up the end of that day's willpower rather than depleting the day's supply before you know when you might need it. Before bed, lay out your clothes for the morning, pack what you need in your bag for the day, maybe even make the decision as to what your most important three tasks are the next day, then go to sleep and let your willpower recharge for tomorrow.

Another important mental change to make is to avoid ruminating and overthinking. Spending mental energy weighing up the decision to attend a party that night in case you're tempted to reach for a drink when you're there is asking for trouble. You'll exhaust your willpower simply thinking about what you're going to do that night rather than saving it up for when the drink is in front of you and you really need to call on it. Make a choice, stick with it – don't deviate. The If–Then exercise mentioned in the last chapter really helps with this (see page 55). Studies have clearly shown that people who use the approach have better self-control when temptation strikes, probably because they don't have to decide how to behave in the moment when willpower might be low[50].

Despite all this, you shouldn't be afraid of testing your willpower, I'm aware this might seem to contradict everything above but think of willpower as being like a muscle during exercise – working it fatigues it in the short term and while it's tired it won't perform as well as before – but then it comes back stronger. If you're reading this book a few weeks before you start your month off, testing your willpower daily from now on can prime it and ensure it's working at full capability when your month starts. You don't have to do anything dramatic like quit smoking or train to run a marathon to do this, instead, try setting yourself a simple task to do every day – perhaps flossing your teeth after brushing, getting off the bus two stops early so you walk for ten minutes or eating a piece of fruit each day. Even better, do something a bit unusual like trying to eat your dinner with the wrong hand. Not only does this train willpower, it actually teaches your brain to pause before acting – allowing you to get control of your unconscious thoughts. And that can make you more likely to pause before you reach for a drink.

Willpower is also boosted if you find pleasure in what you are doing. According to a study at the University of Toronto, Canada, if you can turn whatever you're trying to resist into something you want to do – rather than something you feel you should do, it actually gives your self-control a boost and you're more likely to complete your goal or a specific task[51]. So, that list of all the benefits you're going to get from not drinking I keep telling you to make – this is another one of those times to get it out and refer to it. Visualise how great you'll feel tomorrow morning when you realise you've ticked off another successful day in your month or see yourself waking up the morning with a smile on your face because you don't have a hangover.

Finally, language plays a role. When it comes to making a change, tell yourself you can do it: Not *I* can do it – *You* can do it. According to a study by researchers at the US's University of Illinois at Urbana-Champaign speaking about ourselves in the second person increases our ability to stick at something. The researchers suspect it's because it makes us feel as if we're being encouraged by someone else – perhaps a parent, teacher or mentor – and we like to please others, whereas we might not be so willing to put ourselves first[52]. It might also help to rebrand the word willpower itself. I don't think I have any willpower, I was sure I'd have been one of the children who stared at the marshmallow for 14 minutes then, just as the researcher was unwrapping my second treat I'd scoff it. However, while writing this chapter I realised that's not true. It takes willpower every day for me to meet my morning work deadline – and then stay at work to start my next job rather than run gleefully to the beach or the shops. It takes willpower to run long distances when you're in pain – and I've done two marathons. But I don't count on what I call on in those situations willpower – I call it determination. Realising that all I've got to do is channel that determination towards another source makes breaking bad habits seem considerably more doable. In other words, you might want to use commitment, resolve, self-control, backbone, moxie, courage, fortitude, grit ... whatever works for you.

All of the above tips help build willpower to ensure you have supplies to draw on when you need it and there's one final thing to remember: while willpower can get very low, you never completely run out. There's always a little bit left to call on when we need it and what summons that up is motivation. In trials at the State University of New York in Albany, people told they would be paid to carry on with a task they were tiring of and thinking of quitting found enough willpower to keep going and collect the money[53]. If you're struggling summoning willpower at any point, call upon your motivation for sticking with things and allow that desire to reach into your supplies and pull out those last reserves.

Cravings – the nemesis of willpower

Cravings are the sudden, overwhelming desire to consume something. They're very specific in their characteristics – they hit quickly, they are oddly specific and if you give in to your desire, you often feel guilty or regretful afterwards. While we most commonly associate cravings with food, we can have them for alcohol too. In fact, the more you drink the more likely this is as alcohol actually alters the way neurons in the brain behave.

You can divide the cells in the brain into two types – first are the D1 neurons – also known as 'go neurons' that, when stimulated, drive you to make you want to do something, then there're D2 neurons aka 'stop' neurons that are involved with self-control. Recent research from Texas A&M University in the US has shown that alcohol actually changes the shape of D1 neurons in a way that means they are more readily stimulated, making you more likely to crave a drink[54]. On top of this, alcohol also affects the frontal lobe of the brain, the part involved with sensible thought and making the right decisions. Exactly what this means for self-control researchers are only speculating but they think this is why alcohol can be even harder to give up than many other pleasurable things.

The important thing to know though is that cravings don't last long – they normally pass within about 15 minutes. One thing that gets you through that long without ending up with a glass in your hand can be willpower, but if levels are low, it might also be handy to know a couple of other craving busting tactics.

The first is to use mental distraction: the brain can't think of two things at once. If you distract it with positive thoughts, it can't focus on that little voice telling you 'go on, have a vodka and tonic'. You can think of anything you like to bust a craving, but try thinking about the place in which you're happiest. According to research by Canada's McGill University, this worked better than other distraction techniques like trying to remember the alphabet backwards[55], probably because it delivers the brain a reward. If that's not working for you though then simply physically remove yourself from the vicinity of whatever it is that you're craving. Studies at the University of Exeter found that taking a 15 minute walk was enough to stop cravings for chocolate in their tracks – and it's likely to work with alcohol too.

So, there you go – you know why you're quitting, you've learnt how to break habits, you've learnt how to build willpower and you've got a heap of strategies that allow you to cope when you're staring temptation in the face – but before you sign up for your month of choice and enjoy the new teetotal you, there's one more thing to address. While the majority of the effects of giving up alcohol are positive, a few negatives may crop up. The good news is, if you're prepared for them, they're unlikely to derail your plans – the next chapter helps you get prepared.

CHAPTER FIVE

Handling the Hiccups

Hiccups are the small bumps in the road that might occur while you're quitting booze. Some of these are minor health side effects that may occur when you stop drinking alcohol; others are feelings you might normally use alcohol to tackle and which you need to find alternative solutions for now. The last 'hiccup' group are simply situations you might have to contend with while you're not drinking, and which it's good to plan for.

If you are prepared for these problems it's extremely unlikely that they will be the thing that stops you making it to the end of the month. That's why they're called hiccups – they're a bit annoying but nothing to really worry about. Think of this chapter as the sobriety equivalent of learning how to drink a glass of water while trying to hold your breath!

Disturbed Sleep

While sleep usually improves when you quit drinking, if you normally rely on a nightcap to help you drop off, the opposite might occur and you might find it hard to sleep. The main reason for this is that you're now relying on your own body to send you to sleep rather than the sedative effect of alcohol and, if you have a busy mind or a slightly disrupted body clock, this might not happen as naturally as you might hope. Some simple tweaks can help improve things though.

To fall asleep we need to produce a hormone called melatonin, which is released naturally as the day gets darker. The problem is many of us are disrupting our production of this by exposing our body to blue light from devices like tablets or smartphones in the evening. If you're having trouble dropping off and regularly use gadgets at night, the first thing you need to do is reduce this effect with what experts call an electric sundown. At least four hours before bed, turn the brightness on any devices as far down as you can and hold your device at least 35 cm (14 inches) away from your face, which limits melatonin suppression[56]. One hour before bed however, that's it – everything electronic goes off to put your body into the optimum state for sleep.

It will also help to ensure your bedroom is ready for you to sleep. To sleep well your bedroom needs to be three things … dark, quiet and cool. Here's how to prepare things well.

Darkness

Get into bed at your normal bedtime and turn off the lights. Instead of closing your eyes though allow them to adjust to the dark and look around, what can you see? In the perfect bedroom you should be able to see shapes of things like furniture but no real details. If you put a book in front of your face and can read the type it's definitely too light in there. If you can clearly see obvious bright light from outside the house then use darker curtains to block this. If the glow is inside, for example from a clock radio or charging cell phone, then move that item out of the room.

Quiet

Noise can be very disruptive to sleep – even if you don't realise it. A study published in the European Heart Journal found that sounds of over 35 decibels (equivalent to a car going past) increased blood pressure levels when people were asleep, showing it was disturbing their rest even though they didn't actually wake up[57]. The problem with noise like traffic, trains or music from the neighbours is twofold – it's often not constant which disturbs you and it's also not under your control which can trigger a stress response that makes it harder to sleep. If this sounds like your environment, adding a constant noise like a white noise machine or bedroom fan can block things out. It might sound counterintuitive to add noise to fight noise, but because it's a constant sound under your control it's more likely to be soothing than stressful.

Temperature

Our temperature naturally falls before we fall asleep and rises to wake us up, so a hot room that prevents this fluctuation is more likely to lead to a lighter sleep. The perfect bedroom temperature is 15–20°C (59–68°F) so adjust heating and bedding accordingly. At very least, if it's chilly out then put on some socks. According to researchers from the Psychiatric University Clinic in Basel Switzerland we fall asleep more quickly if our feet are warm as it dilates blood vessels in the area, which lowers internal temperature helping us drop off[58].

One thing not to do is take sleeping pills. Try not to replace the crutch of alcohol with one of medication. The average person taking a sleeping pill falls asleep only 13 minutes faster – and feels worse the next day than if they hadn't taken anything to help[59]. You can however naturally promote melatonin production by drinking a 200 ml glass of tart cherry juice morning and night. According to studies at the US's Louisiana State University, this increased the amount of time insomniacs slept by an impressive 85 minutes[60]. Cherry Active is a good brand to look out for.

The above tips will help stimulate the biological processes that lead to sleep, but for the best results you might also need to train your brain to switch off. There's something about a quiet, dark room with no distractions that means our brains love to start working – everything you've got to do in life, everything you're worried about, it'll all appear about five minutes after you try to go to sleep. Focus on these thoughts and you'll create a state of arousal that keeps you awake. When this happens many people also start to worry about the fact that they aren't sleeping, which adds to the arousal further; this is the process that starts to turn a bad night's sleep into insomnia.

The solution, according to the latest theory in sleep medicine, is to accept what's going on rather than trying to fight it. So, as you lie there, instead of focusing on your thoughts or panicking that you need to get up in a few hours, you accept that your brain is being a bit overactive right now and just chill out about it. Now divert your thoughts to a more calming pattern using mindfulness.

Mindfulness is the idea of living completely in the now rather than thinking about the past or worrying about the future. There are a lot of techniques that help you practise it but one of the most popular is also one of the easiest to do when lying in bed at night and it's called the Five Senses exercise.

Five Senses Exercise

In this exercise, you focus on each of your five senses slowly in turn – you don't react to what you sense, you just notice it and let it go. It doesn't matter what order you work in – just spend a minute or two focusing on each.

Hearing

Notice the sounds around you. Focus on internal sounds like your breathing or the sound of your heart beating or hear what's around you – a ticking clock, the sounds of wind outside or even traffic going past. Remember, don't judge the sound, don't think of it as good or bad, just notice that it's there.

Smell

Can you smell anything around you – the scent of the oil you used at bath time, the book by your bedside table, your partner's perfume or aftershave? Again, don't judge the smell – it doesn't matter if you can still smell the food you cooked for dinner, it'll pass. Just notice what's there.

Sight

If you followed the sleep hygiene tips above, your bedroom should be fairly dark, but that's okay, close your eyes and simply observe the darkness – you might find some colours playing across your eyelids – again, don't wonder about these, just observe them.

Taste

Can you taste anything right now – maybe the mint of the toothpaste you brushed your teeth with before bed?

Touch

Feel yourself sinking into the bed; notice the coolness of the pillow against your face, the lightness of the sheets or heaviness of the blankets on your body. Work up muscle by muscle – chances are, by the time you reach your head you'll be asleep.

If the above alone doesn't help, investigate the books and app of sleep specialist Dr Guy Meadows (thesleepschool. org). He's helped thousands of chronic insomniacs overcome their problems with his 'acceptance' based approach to sleeping.

Drunken People

One thing you realise when you're the sober one at a table full of merry folk is that drunken people can actually be rather annoying. They have a tendency to repeat themselves, they touch you more than you might think is appropriate and boy, can they be loud! If you're going to go out with people who are drinking during your month off you need strategies so they won't drive you mad.

One way to handle this is to leave when things start getting messy – at this point, don't go round saying goodbye to all concerned. Perhaps tell one, more sober, friend that you're leaving just so people don't worry about you, but otherwise just slip quietly out of the door so you don't have to try and justify your departure.

It's also helpful to know what type of drunk people become: According to the University of Missouri-Columbia there are four types of drunk – some of them you won't mind spending time with when you're sober, others are best avoided[61]. The researchers broke them down into personalities they named after famous individuals or characters ...

Hemingways: these are people who act pretty much the same drunk or sober. They always get home and rarely get into any trouble – about 42 per cent of the people studied fell into this group and they are good sober drinking buddies. Mary Poppins are friendly drunks who just like to have fun under the influence. They account for around 15 per cent of drinkers and are also good company most of the night – although they will end up telling you they love you at 2am. Then there're the 20 per cent of people who turn into Nutty Professors – the person dancing on the table or wearing a cone on their head after they've had a few – whether they are the life and soul of the party or your absolute nightmare might depend on what mood you're in when you encounter them. And finally, there're the 23 per cent of the population studied that researchers named Mr Hyde – these are the ones who turn into another person when they are drunk. They might become aggressive, weepy, less sensible or just a pain in the butt – these you definitely want to avoid if you're sober (and maybe, afterwards too!).

Handling Friends and Partners

Not drinking can be seen as an odd behaviour to others – they might think you'll be less fun than normal, or be afraid that they can't indulge in alcohol because you're not. Some drinkers don't like to drink alone and as such might even be slightly angry that your choice is impacting on how they feel they can behave. They might even spend a lot of time and effort attempting to get you to change your mind – meaning you're going to expend willpower staying on the straight and narrow. All of this can make your sober month a bit trying on some relationships.

In some instances you'll know who is going to not take your decision well, and the best advice is to try and avoid them during this month if at all possible. If that's impossible though then use disguise – carry a wine glass with cranberry juice in it or order a non-alcoholic beer and pour it into a glass so no one realises – unless the person concerned is actually going to buy you a drink they won't necessarily register what's in the glass. If they do offer to buy you a drink then say 'Actually, can I just have lemonade this round,' and style it out. Or tell the truth, but be confident in your choice – don't apologise for what you're doing, just state that this month you aren't drinking and that you'll just have lemonade (or whatever your choice is). Don't get defensive or confrontational, just smile and say 'I'm good with lemonade right now,' and keep repeating it. Remember, their reaction to this situation is their issue not yours. Your concern is reaching the end of the month booze free.

If you know none of this is going to work, then lie! There are a few excuses that people are more likely to class as acceptable reasons for not drinking so use them. They include …

- I'm going to the doctor in the morning
- I'm having a blood test tomorrow
- I'm on antibiotics
- I'm still hungover from last night
- I actually feel a bit sick/have a headache
- I'm driving (only to be used on people who live nowhere near you)
- I'm training for a marathon (this generally works best if you don't see the person that often otherwise you might actually have to run said marathon).

The good thing is that as more and more people sign up for schemes like Dry January or Dryathlon, it becomes far more acceptable than it once was to take a break and so at some point you might find you don't need to battle your friends during your month off. Women also have an advantage here – say you're not drinking and everyone will just assume you're pregnant and not ready to tell anyone yet.

Headaches

In the first day or two after quitting you might actually wake up feeling slightly hungover – a bit headachy and jittery. This is most common in regular drinkers and is actually a sign of very slight withdrawal and should be a wake-up call that this month off is exactly what you need to be doing. The aches will pass in a day or two, but in the meantime, a simple painkiller like aspirin or paracetamol can help. Also, keep up your fluid intake. While it's true that alcohol triggers dehydration, if you drink larger drinks like pints of lager you're also consuming a fair amount of fluid and if you take that out of your diet and don't replace it with non-alcoholic liquid you might find you actually end up slightly dehydrated. A good sign to tell if you're adequately hydrated is to check the colour of your urine – it should be a light lemon colour. If it's darker, have a glass of water or a soda.

Lack of confidence

The idea that alcohol raises confidence is so ingrained in society there's even a phrase for it – Dutch Courage. Exactly where this phrase comes from no one knows – there're stories about soldiers swigging Dutch gin before going in to battle or Dutch captains plying their sailors with brandy before fights. No one has verified the true origin, yet that doesn't stop many of us believing in it. If you're one of them and commonly have a drink to raise your confidence before certain situations it can seem harder to face them during your month sober.

But what if I said you didn't need alcohol to feel confident? That actually it's just as likely that your bravery was created by your mind? That was the conclusion of a French study that aimed to find out if alcohol really does raise confidence. In the study, researchers at the University of Grenoble gave two groups of people a tasty (non-alcoholic) fruit drink[62]. One group was told the drink had alcohol in it, one was told it was alcohol-free. All the drinkers were then asked to do a speech and rate how well they thought they'd done afterwards. In every case, those who thought they'd had alcohol rated themselves higher than those who thought their drink had been non-alcoholic, even though both groups had drunk the same thing! Their confidence boost had come not from alcohol, but what's known as the placebo effect where we perceive something has improved, even though there's no real reason for it to happen. The upshot of this is that chances are you'd be just as confident without your drink as you are with it, even more so in fact, as your brain is completely unimpaired.

Saying that though, it can be daunting to walk into a party or work event where you don't know anyone so here's some tips that can help make you feel more comfortable …

1. Get to any event early. Most shy people get to an event late, but this makes it more likely that you'll have to break into established groups and conversations. Get there early and you'll be the person people gravitate to. If you do have to approach people though, look for people with rounded features. According to the theory of face reading, round features – like wide eyes, full lips,

plump cheeks – signify a welcoming friendly person who'll be happy to chat to you, making you feel like a social success from the start.

2. Stand with your back to something solid. According to the Chinese art of Feng Shui this is an important way to feel supported and stable. If nerves start to strike turn your attention to your feet – feeling them solidly on the floor can ground you and boost confidence.

3. Investigate. If you're nervous about starting party conversations, do some research before you head out to create some conversation starters. Maybe find out a bit about the venue it is being held in – find out its history or if it's a restaurant learn a few things about the chef or their signature dish. It's also good to think of questions around general newsy subjects like new films that are out or (non-controversial) headlines. Asking other people's opinions on these means you don't have to know everything about the subject to start a conversation – and lets others who might enjoy being the centre of attention more take the floor.

4. Stand tall. The higher the level of testosterone in your system the more confident you feel and a simple way to raise levels is to stand like Wonder Woman. Put your hands on your hips, spread your feet hip-width apart and throw your shoulders back. Studies have shown that this helps raise testosterone, lowers the stress hormone cortisol that aggravates nerves and actually makes people feel more powerful[63].

5. Notice someone's eye colour. Making eye contact with someone makes them think you're more confident, but it

can be hard to do if you're shy so instead make it a rule to notice everyone's eye colour as you meet them. You'll then look them in the eye in the crucial first seconds when they'll form their opinion of you – but it won't feel as uncomfortable as actually trying to 'make eye contact' might.

Special Occasions

If it's someone's wedding during your month of abstinence or your best friend announces she's just got engaged then you may want to give yourself a pass out and just enjoy the evening and go back on the wagon the next day. If you're doing one of the official challenges you can now even buy a Golden Ticket that gives you a pass out in return for an extra contribution to the charity you're choosing to support – although, if you're buying one every Saturday night it's probably not in the spirit of things. Weddings and engagement and birthday parties are acceptable use of a Golden Ticket; a normal Saturday night at the White Horse not so much! The key point if you use a pass out though is that you get right back on board your mission the next day.

But if you do really want to stick at things, no problem! This is the time to turn to the 50 tips in Chapter Two (see page 30) to get you through the night with your sobriety intact. The night before the party, go back over the list and decide on the ten tactics you think are going to work best for you that night. However, you must not regret your decision and mope around sulking that you're not on the Prosecco with everyone else. Remember, you've actively made a choice to stick on your month off – that's the choice you want to make and the one that makes you feel good about yourself – therefore there's no need to feel down about it. Dance, smile, laugh, throw yourself toward the bouquet and enjoy yourself – after all, it's the occasion and the celebration that should be providing the fun, not what's in your glass.

Stress

It's true that alcohol does help reduce feelings of stress. It dampens activity in your central-nervous system, slows your breathing and heart rate, reduces the mental chatter that creates havoc in your brain, and in doing all of this it calms. No wonder we turn to it when we're stressed but this is also why overwork is one of the biggest lifestyle traits associated with heavy drinking and why people working 55 hours a week or longer are 12 per cent more likely to be heavy drinkers than those working fewer than 48 hours a week[64].

But alcohol isn't a healthy solution to stress; it merely masks the symptoms without you ever tackling what's causing it. And that's bad news as stress is harmful for the body. When you're stressed, blood pressure goes up, the heart beats faster, your muscles tense leading to aches and pains and you trigger a state of inflammation that actively ages the body and which is now being linked to all manner of disease. Rather than masking stress, its far better to try and tackle it, and this month gives you the perfect opportunity to do so.

Discussing every approach that can help fight stress would take another book, so instead, let's focus here on the most important idea – changing the way you think.

A lot of the stress in our lives is created in our own heads as we worry about what might happen in a given situation. Imagine the scenario of two people on a train on the way to a meeting. The train stops and an announcement comes over the loudspeaker explaining that, due to a broken down train ahead, they are going to be stuck here a while. At this point Person One starts to stress, in their head their thoughts start to whirl – they're going to miss the meeting, their boss will be furious, redundancies are planned, this is it, the deciding factor – they're going to lose their job. The whole journey is miserable and even though they do get there on time the stress has affected how well they perform. Person Two thinks, 'Oh here we go, another late train.' They get on their phone, call the people they are meeting to explain they are going to be late, find out they are stuck on the train behind and will be even later. They spend the rest of the journey feeling relaxed and ace the meeting. The same scenario, two very different outcomes – how you think about stress is absolutely related to how intensely you feel it – so, work on your thinking …

Schedule Worry Time

Allow 20–30 minutes once a day to tackle worries; if concerns appear at other points during the day write them on a list and tell yourself you'll tackle them during worry time – by the time you reach your scheduled 20 minutes most of the things you were worried about will no longer be relevant.

Think positive

When we're in a stressed state we tend to develop tunnel vision and often focus only on what we haven't done rather than what we've achieved. Reset your mindset by focusing on positives. Before you go to sleep, or at any other point in the day you find it helpful, spend a few minutes focusing on three things that you are grateful for or that went well today.

Plan properly

If you're always late then there's a good chance you also regularly feel stressed about it. The most common reason people are late is that they simply underestimate how long things will take. So, from now on, when you're deciding how long it's going to take to get somewhere or carry out a task, add at least 40 per cent more time than you think and you could immediately find your stress reduces.

Don't meet your friends to rant

A study from the University of Kent found that ranting to friends about what's wrong with life actually encourages brooding behaviour that makes us more unhappy[65]; spending time constructively thinking about what's wrong and how to solve it gets a much better reaction – and you'll be clear headed enough this month to do it.

Sugar Cravings

Alcohol is made from fermented sugar and some people find that when they stop drinking their body starts to crave the sugar that it's now missing. Sugar also helps replace neurotransmitters like serotonin, dopamine and endorphins normally provided by alcohol.

The diet plan that follows this chapter is specifically designed to help prevent sugar cravings. It uses a healthy mix of low-sugar carbohydrates, fats and proteins to balance blood sugar throughout the day, reducing the peaks and troughs in energy that can set cravings in motion. It also contains foods that support the production of the neurotransmitters your brain is seeking. If cravings do happen I'd strongly suggest trying the diet plan if you haven't already. You can also use the general craving busting tips I talked about in Chapter Four and for some extra help, here's some further advice specifically shown to tackle sugar cravings:

1. Sniff some vanilla oil. Researchers at the UK's St George's Hospital found smelling vanilla helped reduce cravings for sweet treats like chocolate. It's believed it actually stimulates serotonin, improving mood[66].
2. Visualise a rainbow. Or some flowers or a puppy. According to research by Australia's Flinders University, when you crave a particular food you actually picture it in your mind. However, your brain can't think of two things at once, so if you replace the foodie pic with something else, you'll distract yourself out of it[67].

3. Take a magnesium supplement. Low magnesium levels are linked to sugar cravings – particularly those that occur premenstrually in women. Magnesium is also very calming and can help if your cravings are triggered by stress. Women need 270mg a day, men need 300mg.

4. A 500mg capsule of the amino-acid l-glutamine, snapped open and sprinkled on the tongue will stop a sugar binge quickly. L-glutamine converts to glucose in the system and so supplies your body with a quick shot of sugar – but with far fewer calories than half a dozen sweets.

Time to Fill

Going to the pub is an easy night out – there's normally one nearby, you know what you're going to do when you get there and it doesn't normally cost too much. If you're giving up drinking and trying to avoid temptation, you may need to stay home more, and if you don't fill the time with other activities you might find yourself getting bored. This is not something we're really used to doing any more and it can actually be an uncomfortable sensation.

Think about it – when was the last time you literally sat and did nothing. The day has gone when you sat on the bus daydreaming as the world went past the window. Now, with the advent of smartphones we're constantly stimulating our brains and we're not very good at mentally doing nothing. However, our brains need time to recharge and it's been suggested that after a period of boredom we're actually more motivated to make changes and have more creative thoughts. Boredom is also a stimulus for self-reflection – handy at a time when you're supposed to be reassessing your relationship with alcohol and the triggers that cause you to consume it.

As such, there're two solutions to having time on your hands – you can keep busy filling your time with tasks you normally don't have time to do or, more radically, you can embrace your free time – and the feeling of boredom that might come with it. But to do this positively, you need to know what type of boredom you have. There are five types, says experts, and they need handling in different ways[68].

Indifferent boredom

In this type you feel relaxed and calm. Time seems to be dragging, but you're not actively searching for something new to do. It's possible that this type of boredom is good for us – a way of giving our minds and bodies a rest from stimulation. Embrace it, stare out the window, look at the ceiling and just let your thoughts wander wherever they need to go.

Apathetic boredom

This is not an enjoyable feeling; it's associated with low mood and feeling of helplessness – your time might be your own, but you don't feel like you have a choice what to do with it. If this type of boredom strikes, do something you know makes you happy – listen to an album you haven't heard since your teens, watch a film that always makes you smile, head out for a walk somewhere beautiful. Or do something for others. The positive mental lift this gives us is particularly good for tackling this type of boredom.

Calibrating boredom

Your mind is wandering, you know you want to do something different but you aren't sure what. A good solution to this type of boredom is to call a friend. People with calibrating boredom are very susceptible to trying new things or ideas that are suggested to them so get your buddy to suggest something and head out and do it. Just make sure you pick the friend who isn't going to suggest you go the pub!

Reactant boredom

This jittery form of boredom means the lack of something to do makes you frustrated and anxious. It's good to try and break out of this type of boredom as it's believed to have negative effects on our health. Something physical might particularly help here as it releases that jittery sensation allowing you to think more clearly and find what you really want to do with your time.

Searching boredom

You're feeling restless but not angry or frustrated – you know you want to do something new, you just need to find what it is. Spend the next 10 minutes writing down 20 things you could do now to pass the time – stick a pin in it and do whatever task you choose.

Social exclusion

This was the one negative thing the journalists in the *New Scientist* trial (see page 11) pinpointed during their month off – they didn't see friends as often. Perhaps there were some social occasions they simply didn't feel they could join in without alcohol or maybe some friends didn't invite them out. Remember, having sober people around can be quite difficult for some people to handle.

There're a couple of ways to tackle social exclusion – you can corral your friends into social activities that don't involve alcohol; you can catch up with people by phone or you can use this month as a good excuse to go and find some new friends. I'm not suggesting you dump your nearest and dearest forever but, if you're seriously committing yourself to reducing alcohol in the longer term it'll be good to find some friends who have interests over and above going to the pub. So, visit friend-finding sites like meetup.com and find groups who want to go to the cinema or like walking or simply choose groups that meet at coffee houses or other dry venues. Or just hang out with pregnant friends! They can't drink for nine months – your thirty days is nothing in comparison.

Joking aside, with these plans to handle the most common hiccups you might encounter during your month off then it's likely that you now have every tactic in place for success. You're pretty much ready to go now but before you start, you might want to take a trip to the supermarket. What you eat can help support how great you feel during your month off, it can boost how easy success is to achieve – and can increase the chance of you achieving any weight loss goals. The next chapter explains what to do and gives a diet plan you can follow to achieve it.

CHAPTER SIX

The Craving-Busting Diet Plan

When you give up drinking you might notice a few changes in your appetite. You'll notice it's far easier to eat healthily. You're not tempted by late night diet-blowing snacks or morning-after hangover munchies – however, on the flip side, you might develop sugar cravings as your body tries to replace the buzz it gets from alcohol via alternative sweet foods. You could also find that when you're not spending your evenings drinking you need other sensory pleasures to feel satisfied, which can see you nibbling a bit more than you should. Getting the balance right between these effects will help maximise the chances that your month off ends up in weight loss, not weight gain.

This is where this diet plan comes in. First up, it is calorie controlled which powers your weight loss goals. Despite this though, it's packed with tasty food combinations and indulgent dishes like curry, sausage and mash and burgers that mean you won't feel deprived of comforting food while you're focusing on quitting alcohol.

But it also specifically stabilises blood sugar levels to help you fight cravings and it contains foods that are likely to further increase your chance of success by promoting positive thinking, better moods and a healthier reaction to stress. Let me explain ...

All carbs are not evil

One main job of this plan is help stabilise your blood sugar levels to minimise the sugar cravings that might see you turning to alcohol. The best way to do this is to eat a balanced mix of protein foods like meat, fish, eggs and dairy, fat from foods like avocado, oily fish, nuts, seeds and healthy oils and some healthy carbohydrates.

Yes, carbohydrates. You will consume pasta, bread, crackers and other carb-based goodies of excitement this month. A lot of diets nowadays ban carbohydrates and while it can be a very effective way to reduce weight very quickly, it requires a lot of willpower to stay focused – willpower that right now you should be spending on staying away from alcohol. As such, this plan includes carbs, but it chooses the right ones – those referred to as low GI carbs.

GI stands for glycemic index and it's a measure of how fast a food turns into the sugar glucose in your body. Glucose is the body's preferred source of fuel and it makes it from the starches and sugars in the food we eat. However, while we need glucose, we need it in steady measured doses and the body works hard to stabilise how much is in the bloodstream at any one time. If too much is released too quickly, the body shuttles the excess into the fat stores which not only adds extra pounds on the scales, but also triggers a rollercoaster type pattern of energy where one hour you're buzzing but the next, your energy and mood are in your boots and you're desperate for something sweet – this craving can easily manifest as a need for a drink. Eat so that your glucose – aka blood sugar – level is stable and you'll find you have more balanced energy, more stable mood, fewer sugar and alcohol cravings, greater willpower and you may find it easier to maintain – or even lose – weight.

The GI of a food is determined by a couple of different factors – predominantly whether it contains carbohydrate or not. Foods that are made solely of protein like meat and fish automatically have a low GI as do foods like butter or avocado that contain large amounts of fat. Within carbohydrate foods, however, the more fibre a carbohydrate contains the slower it digests and the lower its GI; conversely if a food contains a lot of starch, particularly processed forms of starch like you find in many breakfast cereals or flour the body digests it faster and so its GI is higher. The type of sugar a food contains also plays a role – foods containing a lot of glucose have a high GI. Sucrose, the type found in table sugar, converts to glucose moderately quickly and so foods containing mostly sucrose often have a medium GI. Fructose, the main sugar in fruit, and lactose, the main sugar in dairy products, convert more slowly and so these foods have either a low or moderate GI. Mixes of protein and carbs like beans, pulses and legumes have a lower GI than purely starchy carbs. The good news is, you don't need to work out which of the above characteristics apply to the food you're consuming because scientists have done the maths for you. Here's a quick guide.

Breads

High GI: Bagels, baguettes, gluten-free bread, white bread, roti, naan

Medium GI: Brown bread, chapatti, fruit bread, pitta bread, sourdough, white tortilla wraps, white or brown bread with added fibre

Low GI: Barley, rye or pumpernickel, breads with grains or seeds, corn tortilla, granary bread, soya bread, wheat tortilla wraps

Cereals

High GI: Most flaked cereals, honey-coated cereals, instant porridge, puffed cereals, rice cereals

Medium GI: Bran cereal with fruit, muesli with sugar, wheat cereal

Low GI: Bran noodles like All Bran, porridge oats, sugar-free muesli with nuts/seeds

Grains and legumes

High GI: Millet, amaranth

Medium GI: Couscous, spelt, polenta

Low GI: Barley, bulgur wheat, buckwheat, quinoa, all beans, legumes and pulses

Pasta and noodles

High GI: Gluten-free noodles

Medium GI: Soba noodles, udon noodles

Low GI: All pastas, egg noodles, glass noodles, kelp noodles

Potatoes

High GI: Baked, French fries, mash

Medium GI: Crisps, sweet potatoes, gnocchi

Low GI: New potatoes, yams

Rice

High GI: Fast-cook varieties, jasmine rice, sticky rice, sushi rice

Medium GI: Basmati, brown rice, microwave rices, risotto, white rice

Low GI: The only low GI rice is an Australian variety called Doongara. It's not sold readily in the UK yet.

Balancing your brain chemicals

Eating a balanced diet based around fresh, natural foods is key when it comes to creating the positive mental attitude you need to change habits and stick to a goal. All of the main food groups – aka macronutrients – play a role in keeping levels of the chemicals we need for positive mental health balanced. Protein foods like meat, fish, eggs, dairy and beans are good sources of the amino acid l-tyrosine that your body needs to synthesise the reward hormone dopamine. Wholegrain carbohydrates contain B vitamins that you need to help the body handle stress plus carbohydrates are involved with the production of serotonin, the neurotransmitter that controls mood. And as for fat, it's important for optimum brain function, it helps slow down how fast meals are digested leading to a more balanced blood sugar and it helps keep you fuller for longer, which can help reduce cravings.

Within these macronutrients though, there are also some specific foods that can help support the brain while you quit alcohol and the diet that follows also includes plenty of these to boost results. They include …

Blueberries

Neurogenesis is the scientific name for building new brain cells. A brain in which there is high neurogenesis finds it easier to cope with stress. Blueberries are also high in vitamin C and research from Germany's University of Trier has shown we calm down faster from stress if vitamin C levels in the body are high[69].

Chilli peppers

Endorphins are the substances released during exercise that create the so-called 'runner's high', which makes exercisers feel so energised and positive. Chilli peppers also trigger endorphin release. And they raise metabolism and lower appetite, which can boost results if you're hoping to lose weight during your month off.

Dark green vegetables like spinach, kale or broccoli

Low levels of the B vitamin folate are associated with poor mood and depression, and dark green vegetables are good sources of folate. On top of this, spinach, kale, cabbage and parsley also contain l-glutamine, an amino acid thought to decrease cravings for sugar and alcohol. Cooking destroys this, though which is why you'll find a lot of salad-based options using these foods in the plan.

Fermented foods

These help top up levels of the bacteria that live in our gut and right now there's a lot of evidence pointing to these bugs playing an important role in reducing the impact of stress and anxiety. It seems that the bacteria produce chemicals that actively calm us and improve mood – for example, when the bacteria break down carbohydrates they create a fatty acid called butyrate which increases levels of the mood booster serotonin in the body. Simply eating a yoghurt containing four specific strains of bacteria twice a day caused people to react more calmly to stress in one trial at the US's University of California Los Angeles. Fermented foods include natural yoghurt, sauerkraut, kimchi, miso soup and pickles.

Oily fish

It's a great source of healthy omega-3 fats. These are vital generally for good brain health but they have also been specifically shown to help build resilience to stress. In Australian research, students taking an omega-3 supplement during exams were less stressed by the process than those who hadn't taken supplements[70]. Omega-3 fats also contain substances that help slow the breakdown of dopamine in the brain; this helps keep your levels of the reward chemical high.

Pumpkin seeds

These provide tryptophan, an amino acid that's needed to make several important hormones involved with the regulation of mood. Notably, tryptophan helps create serotonin – the neurotransmitter most involved with feeling more positive and the B vitamin niacin, which can help reduce risk of depression. It also helps you produce the sleep hormone melatonin

Turmeric

This bright yellow spice is what gives curries their intense colour. It's known for improving overall brain health, but it also helps improve mood as it naturally increases levels of a substance in the brain called BDNF. Low levels of this are clearly linked to depression – in fact, one way anti-depressants work is to raise BDNF levels. Obviously, you can cook with turmeric, but if you don't have time to cook from scratch every day, start your day with a turmeric tea (Pukka Herbs sell a good one), whip up a turmeric latte or try a supplement.

How to use the diet plan

Following this plan is not an essential part of quitting alcohol – in fact, some experts would say if you're really concerned that your month off is going to be tough, changing your diet as well could be a bad idea as it will use up some of your willpower. Looking at it another way though, the fact that meals here are set out for you does give you three fewer decisions to make each day.

If you do want to follow the plan, it couldn't be easier – simply pick one meal each for breakfast, lunch and dinner. All the meals are simple and easy to prepare and you can carry the lunches to work fairly easily. There's a panel of ready-to-buy suggestions if that suits you better, and a panel of suggested snacks for when you're peckish.

You'll notice a lot of recipes in the plan. This is because stimulating your tastebuds with interesting tastes and textures can help make up for the lack of alcohol during you month off, but don't worry if you don't like cooking or don't have time to cook in the week as for any meal where there's a recipe, there's also an alternative option that's quicker to prepare. Remember though, embracing home cooking is a healthy way to fill evenings normally spent at the pub so you're not getting away with just popping something in the microwave here!

Because so many people hope to lose weight when they give up alcohol, the plan contains smaller portions of higher calorie foods that can help boost these results. If you're not specifically aiming for weight loss, feel free to ignore the suggested portion sizes and simply eat to your appetite.

If you don't like a meal or ingredient on the plan, that's okay – simply repeat a meal from another day. There's no magic formula here that means you won't get the benefits if you swap something round. It's also okay to swap like-for-like if you don't like something or simply want to use things up. I've given lots of different suggestions each week to ensure the diet is varied, but if you're just cooking for one or two I know how annoying it is to have half a head of broccoli left over from Monday going off in the fridge because Tuesday's meal plan says to eat cabbage and Wednesday's vegetable is carrots – so feel free to repeat things, change vegetables for other vegetables, swap in a different meat or fish. Or if you're vegetarian, use tofu, eggs or dairy instead of meat. If you don't have quinoa feel free to use pasta. Work to what's in your fridge and your shopping budget.

The only rules you must follow are that most of the carbohydrates you eat must be low or medium GI and that highly refined carbohydrates like white bread and sugary snacks or treats are banned. Also, try to keep in a good selection of the brain-boosting foods mentioned above. You can also add more of the low-calorie forms of these if you like – use extra chilli, turmeric or parsley to flavour meals or add an extra portion of dark leafy greens.

Right, enough theory, let's show you what eating to fight cravings actually looks like ...

The One-Month Craving-Busting Plan

Day 1

You're motivated, you're focused, you're raring to go. That's great – get to it. If, however, you're a bit sceptical about your ability to do this, concentrate only on not drinking today using whatever tactics it takes from the last few chapters to make that happen. Tomorrow decide to do exactly the same thing, then simply repeat until the month is over and ta da – you've quit drinking for a month. If this sounds like you, today's Must Do is to clear all alcohol from the house – throw it away, give it away, lock it in a box and keep the key at the office – whatever. If there's no alcohol in the house it means you'll have to make a considered effort to have a drink rather than reaching for one on autopilot. And that gives you a chance to make a different choice.

Breakfast: Two slices of toasted sourdough bread topped with a quarter of an avocado, mashed. Top with one poached egg.

Lunch: Salad of spinach, tomato, red onion and 60 g (2¼ oz) smoked salmon or 50 g (2 oz) grilled halloumi cheese. Add 5–6 black olives and 1 tablespoon of oil and vinegar.

Dinner: Tandoori Chicken with Minted Quinoa (see recipe on page 136).

Alternative: 1 ready-to-eat flavoured chicken fillet (around 125 g/4½ oz) or a Quorn Steak with 50 g (2oz) (dry weight) quinoa made as directed. Add chopped tomato and cucumber a little chopped fresh mint.

Day 2

Breakfast: 40 g (1½ oz) steel-cut porridge oats prepared as directed with 125 ml (4½ fl oz) milk. Two or three handfuls of blueberries.

Lunch: Salad of fresh kale and celery tossed in 1 tablespoon Caesar dressing. Add 3–4 fresh anchovies if you like them and top with 100 g (4 oz) grilled chicken or 150 g (5 oz) cottage cheese. 1 slice of toasted sourdough.

Dinner: 125 g (4½ oz) lamb chop, grilled, or a 70 g (2½ oz) slice of nut roast. Serve with 150 g (5 oz) boiled new potatoes, a portion of green beans and 1–2 tablespoons sauerkraut (you can buy this in many supermarkets now but pick a brand that is fermented by salting rather than pickling). Add some mint sauce or a little gravy if you like.

Day 3

Breakfast: Turmeric Latte (see recipe on page 131) or a cup of turmeric tea. Two oatcake style biscuits served with 1 teaspoon each peanut butter. Any piece of fruit.

Lunch: Salad of watercress or spinach with 150 g (5 oz) boiled new potatoes, 2 boiled eggs, chopped tomato and cucumber. Top with a little mustard mixed with vinegar.

Dinner: Salmon Fishcakes (see recipe on page 138) served with broccoli and carrots.

Alternative: One pre-made large salmon fishcake or a veggie burger. Served with 200 g (7 oz) jacket potato, broccoli and carrots.

Day 4

Time for a benefit audit. You should already be noticing some of the sleep-related benefits of quitting drinking; if you're not, you might have been using alcohol to kick start your sleep process. Start using some of the sleep-boosting tricks on page 77 instead. I also recommend the Aromatherapy Associates Deep Relax Bath and Shower Oil or Salts – they're like knockout drops! Another benefit you might feel now is improved energy as you avoid the draining effects of hangovers and start to experience the blood-sugar-balancing effects of the diet plan. You might also find your stomach has shrunk – alcohol causes fluid retention and bloating which will often disappear after 2–3 days abstinence. Have you noticed any other positives? Write down as many as you can think of. Focus on the benefits, stay positive and keep going.

Breakfast: 150 g (5 oz) Greek yoghurt with one chopped peach and 25 g (1 oz) pumpkin seeds.

Lunch: Sandwich made from two slices of granary, rye or sourdough bread. Fill with 100 g (4 oz) tuna mixed with a little mayonnaise or 150 g (5 oz) cottage cheese. Stir in 1 tablespoon of sweetcorn and layer on some fresh spinach. Serve with carrot sticks.

Dinner: 50 g (2 oz) dry-weight pasta tossed with a sauce of 4 chopped tomatoes and some chopped onion simmered with a little olive oil, garlic and chilli and 50 g (2 oz) sliced pan-fried chorizo or 200 g (8 oz) black beans.

Day 5

Breakfast: Two pieces of granary or sourdough toast with 1 mashed banana and a handful of blueberries. 125 g (4½ oz) plain or Greek yoghurt.

Lunch: Mexican bowl made from rocket or spinach and topped with 150 g (5 oz) canned black beans, 25 g (1 oz) grated cheese, chopped tomato and red onion and quarter of an avocado mashed with a little lime and fresh chilli. Serve with two oatcakes for scooping.

Dinner: Spiced Quick-Fried Prawns (see recipe on page 139) served with 50 g (2 oz) basmati rice.

Alternative: Stir fry of 125 g (4½ oz) large prawns or tofu/tempeh with broccoli, green pepper and bok choy and a little soy sauce, turmeric and fresh ginger. Serve with 50 g (2 oz) basmati rice.

Day 6

Breakfast: 2 eggs scrambled with 50 g (2 oz) smoked salmon. 1 piece of wholegrain or sourdough toast.

Lunch: 75 g (3 oz) houmous with crudités of red pepper, carrot and celery. 1 small wholemeal pitta bread.

Dinner: 125 g (4½ oz) grilled chicken breast or 50 g (2 oz) cashew nuts, stir-fried with unlimited vegetables served on a bed of 50 g (2 oz) quinoa. Add a little salsa, hot sauce or soy sauce for flavour.

Day 7

One week in: chances are you've already faced at least one social hurdle by now and have started to decide which of the 50 tips in Chapter Two are likely to work best for you. If you haven't done so already, then go through and pick the five or six that speak loudest to you, write them on a piece of paper and put it in your purse or wallet. If willpower wanes when you're out and about refer back to it and implement at least one of the tips. Remember cravings last 15 minutes max – keep yourself occupied and they'll pass.

Breakfast: Baked eggs (see recipe on page 132) with 1 piece of sourdough toast.

Or

2 boiled or poached eggs with 1 slice of granary toast topped with sliced tomatoes.

Lunch: 40 g (1½ oz) brie or another cheese of your choice. 2–3 oatcakes, 1 pear, 5–6 black olives, celery sticks.

Dinner: 125 g (4½ oz) lean steak, grilled or pan-fried, or a chilli made from mixed beans, tomatoes and chilli peppers served with 1 medium-sized baked sweet potato and peas.

Day 8

Breakfast: Smoothie of 1 banana, 150 ml (5 fl oz) milk and 1 tablespoon of oats. Piece of any other fruit.

Lunch: Salad of cos lettuce, sun-dried tomato, beetroot and 20 g (¾ oz) pumpkin seeds, topped with 75 g (3 oz) buffalo mozzarella or feta. Splash with some balsamic vinegar.

Dinner: 50 g (2oz) dry weight pasta topped with a sauce made from 100 g (4 oz) beef or Quorn mince and 100 g (4 oz) sliced mushrooms simmered with 200 g (8 oz) chopped canned tomatoes, garlic, oregano.

Day 9

Breakfast: Turmeric Latte (see recipe on page 131) or a cup of turmeric tea. Fruit salad made from any three fruits and 125 g (4½ oz) plain or Greek yoghurt with 20 g (¾ oz) pumpkin seeds.

Lunch: Small jacket potato topped with 2 tablespoons tuna mayonnaise, chilli, baked beans or coleslaw. Serve with a green salad.

Dinner: Bruschetta of Mushrooms on Wilted Spinach (see recipe on page 140).

Alternative: Grill one large portobello mushroom, served on a bed of sautéed spinach crumbled with 25 g (1 oz) feta cheese. Serve with 1 slice of sourdough bread.

Day 10

Breakfast: Chia Pudding (see recipe on page 133) or buy a ready-made Chia Pod, mixed with two handfuls of any berry and 20 g (3/4 oz) pumpkin seeds.

Lunch: Open sandwich of one slice of rye or granary bread topped with 125 g (4½ oz) smoked mackerel or half an avocado mashed with 1 teaspoon of horseradish. Serve with a salad of rocket and grated beetroot.

Dinner: 125 g (4½ oz) gammon steak, grilled or 1–2 poached eggs. Serve with 125 g (4½ oz) cooked Puy lentils and some leeks cooked in a little butter.

Day 11

I go out a lot and so I've found this is my personal waver point as I'm normally getting fed up with drinking soft drinks. My best motivation now is to think of all the nasty things I've avoided by not drinking – that sense of dread when you open Twitter the morning after, that 'not quite there' feeling the next day that comes after even just one large glass of wine, or the all out horror that is a hangover. I also focus on the fact that when I have given in at this point, I haven't actually enjoyed the drink as much as I thought I would. Thinking negative might work for you too, but if you're more positively focused, instead make a list of all the benefits you've gained so far by not drinking.

Breakfast: Two slices of granary or sourdough toast topped with quarter of avocado, mashed. Add 40 g (1½ oz) smoked salmon or 30 g (1¼ oz) feta, halloumi or other cheese.

Lunch: Small sushi selection box – ideally made with brown rice or quinoa if you can find it. Bowl of miso soup. 1 apple.

Dinner: Spiced Lamb with Spinach and Potato (see recipe on page 142).

Alternative: 125 g (4½ oz) lamb chop or 3–4 falafel balls with 50 g (2 oz) basmati rice and steamed spinach. Add a 1 tablespoon salsa, houmous or gravy.

Day 12

Breakfast: 2 eggs scrambled, poached or boiled with 2 oatcake style biscuits spread with a little butter.

Lunch: Salad of grated carrot, red pepper and watercress topped with a little balsamic dressing. Top with 125 g (4½ oz) of chicken, prawns, salmon or grilled tofu.

Dinner: 125 g (4½ oz) fillet of any white fish, pan fried or a 200 g (8 oz) serving of cauliflower cheese. Serve with 150 g (5 oz) mashed sweet potatoes and some kale.

Day 13

Breakfast: 2 slices of grilled bacon (or one portobello mushroom), 1 poached egg, sliced tomato, spinach.

Lunch: Leek and Potato Soup (see recipe on page 135) or half a 600 ml (1 pint) carton of any fresh vegetable soup. 1 slice of sourdough bread topped with a slice of cheese or 1 teaspoon of soft cheese.

Dinner: 125 g (4½ oz) salmon fillet, or half an aubergine, baked then topped with 50 g (2 oz) feta. Serve with 50 g (2 oz) dry-weight quinoa and green beans.

Day 14

Breakfast: Overnight Oats (see recipe on page 133).

Or

40 g (1½ oz) porridge oats with 125 ml (5 fl oz) natural yoghurt and chopped apple.

Lunch: Wholemeal tortilla-wrap spread with 2 tablespoons mashed black beans. Add salsa, coriander and some fresh chilli and 100 g (4 oz) of fresh prawns or 25 g (1 oz) dry-weight brown rice. Serve with quarter of avocado, mashed, and carrot sticks.

Dinner: Stir-fry of 100 g (3½ oz) lean beef or tofu with yellow peppers, broccoli and cabbage or bok choy cooked in a half a sachet of black bean sauce. Serve with 50 g (2 oz) dry weight of egg noodles.

Day 15

Halfway. That's brilliant! Even if you normally have only one large glass of wine or pint of beer every other night you'll have turned down 18–27 alcohol units (depending on your tipple of choice), cut your calorie intake by over 1,500 calories and saved over £30 at average pub prices. If you drink more a night, or drink more often, the savings and benefits will be even greater. Why not go and celebrate with an alcohol-free night out somewhere you've never been before?

Breakfast: Fruit salad of any three chopped fruit topped with 125 ml (5 fl oz) Greek yoghurt top with 20 g (¾ oz) sprinkle of pumpkin seeds.

Lunch: Pasta salad made from 50 g (2 oz) (dry weight) cooked, cooled pasta. Add 125 g (4½ oz) fresh prawns or 150 g (5 oz) butter beans, some fresh peas and some chopped parsley. Top with lemon juice and mix well.

Dinner: Quarter-pounder burger or a veggie burger, grilled. Top with sliced pickles, onion and lettuce and serve in a wholemeal bap. Add 1–2 tablespoons of sauerkraut

Day 16

Breakfast: Tortilla wrap spread with 1 teaspoon peanut butter and 1 mashed banana. Roll up. Serve with 125 ml (5 fl oz) skimmed milk or a Turmeric Latte (see recipe on page 131).

Lunch: Salad of cos lettuce, chopped celery, chopped apple and 5–6 artichoke hearts served with 60 g (2¼ oz) smoked salmon or one boiled egg and 20 g (¾ oz) pumpkin seeds.

Dinner: Chicken with a Simple Vegetable Stew (see recipe on page 143) served on a bed of 50 g (2 oz) dry weight basmati rice.

Alternative: 125 g (4½ oz) grilled chicken breast or 75 g (3 oz) houmous with unlimited vegetables served on a bed of 50 g (2 oz) dry-weight basmati rice. Add a little salsa, hot sauce or soy sauce for flavour.

Day 17

Breakfast: Overnight Oats (see recipe on page 133).

Lunch: 100 g (4 oz) canned salmon or 150 g (5 oz) cottage cheese served with a salad of cucumber, 1 diced apple and 200 g (8 oz) chickpeas.

Dinner: 50 g (2 oz) – dry weight – pasta served with a sauce of 200 g (8 oz) chopped tomatoes, 5–6 black olives, some garlic and 100 g (3½ oz) canned tuna or 150 g (5 oz) butter beans (or a mix of half each).

Day 18

Breakfast: 40 g (1½ oz) All-Bran-style cereal topped with 125 ml (5 oz) milk and one chopped apple or pear.

Lunch: Leek and Potato Soup (see recipe on page 135) or half a 600 ml (1 pint) carton of any fresh vegetable soup served with a wholemeal roll spread with a little houmous and filled with cucumber and tomato.

Dinner: Asian Beef and Noodles (see recipe on page 145).

Alternative: Stir-fry 100 g (4 oz) beef or tofu with broccoli, mangetout, chilli, ginger and soy sauce. Serve with 50 g (2 oz) dry-weight egg noodles.

Day 19

By now, not ordering alcohol is well on its way to becoming a habit. If you are still finding it a battle of will every day though, then delve deeper into what reward you're missing by not drinking. Remember, part of breaking the alcohol habit is replacing the reward that alcohol gives you – maybe you haven't correctly identified yours yet or you haven't yet found something that gives you the same pleasure. Here're some areas to look at …

- Is the best thing about drinking for you seeing friends? If so, where can you go with them that doesn't revolve around alcohol?
- Do you drink to get out of the house? If so, make a list of other activities that can fill your time.
- Do you like the taste of alcohol? Then swapping for plain water won't satisfy you – try adult soft drinks like Zeo or alcohol-free alternatives like the Sipsmith range designed for a grown-up palette.
- Do you drink to switch off from the day – then, create a new transition ritual instead.

Breakfast: Smoothie of 200 ml (8 fl oz) skimmed milk, 2 handfuls of berries, 25 g (1 oz) oats. Serve with 20 g (¾ oz) of pumpkin seeds.

Lunch: Sandwich of two slices of sourdough or granary bread spread with a little mustard or horseradish. Add 100 g (4 oz) lean roast beef or two boiled eggs, sliced and tomato. Serve with a heaped spoonful of sauerkraut.

Dinner: Grill 125 g (4½ oz) fish fillet (sole, cod, salmon) or a large aubergine baked then topped with 50 g (2 oz) feta cheese and serve with a mixed salad of artichoke hearts, olive, sundried tomato and spinach. Serve with 200 g (8 oz) butter beans, mashed.

Day 20

Breakfast: Savoury Muffin (see recipe on page 134) with a piece of fruit.

Lunch: Three bean salad made from 200 g (8 oz) canned mixed beans with chopped tomato and onion. Add plenty of coriander, lemon juice and a sprinkle of chilli. Serve with 100 g (4 oz) chicken breast or 50 g (2 oz) grilled halloumi.

Dinner: Two pork or vegetarian sausages served with 200 g (8 oz) mashed sweet potato (add a little turmeric if you like) and 150 g (5 oz) peas.

Day 21

Breakfast: 1 poached egg and half an avocado, 1 piece of sourdough or granary toast.

Lunch: 5 falafel balls served with 2 tablespoons houmous, 45–6 olives and a salad of grated carrot and beetroot.

Dinner: Fish Pie with Turmeric Mash (see recipe on page 146). Serve with 1 tablespoon of sauerkraut.

Alternative: 125 g (4½ oz) fillet of salmon, herring or mackerel or a serving of vegetable chilli served with 200 g (7oz) mashed sweet potato served with 1 tablespoon of sauerkraut.

Day 22

Breakfast: Turmeric Latte (see recipe on page 131) 1 apple, 1 pear, 25 g (1 oz) sliced cheese and 1 piece of granary or sourdough bread.

Lunch: Small sushi pack – ideally with brown rice or quinoa if you can get it. Serving of miso soup.

Dinner: 50 g (2 oz) dry-weight risotto rice, made as directed. Mix in 50 g (2 oz) thinly sliced chorizo, pan fried, or 50 g (2 oz) feta cheese, and a few handfuls of mushrooms and chopped asparagus.

Day 23

Spend a while navel gazing. What have you learnt so far about your drinking habits? Where have you found it hardest to resist temptation, which of your friends are happy for you to stay sober, and which haven't taken it well? What soft drink options have you enjoyed most? How have you handled celebrations or setbacks and what can you learn from that? The more you understand your drinking – and any hurdles you've had to overcome – the more tactics you have in place to keep things sensible once you start drinking again.

Breakfast: 40 g (1½ oz) porridge oats made with 125 ml (5 fl oz) milk topped with 1 chopped banana.

Lunch: Salad of kale, asparagus and quarter of an avocado topped with 75 g (3 oz) buffalo mozzarella. 2–3 oatcakes.

Dinner: Chickpeas with Spinach (see recipe on page 148) served on a bed of 50 g (2 oz) quinoa.

Alternative: 200 g (8 oz) chickpeas simmered in 200 g (8 oz) canned tomatoes with a few handfuls of spinach. Add garlic and some chilli. Serve on 50 g (2 oz) quinoa.

Day 24

Breakfast: 200 g (8 oz) Greek yoghurt topped with 1 chopped peach or 2 handfuls of berries, 2 oatcakes crumbled over the top.

Lunch: Egg sandwich made from two slices of granary or rye bread filled with 1 sliced hardboiled egg, a little cress, some fresh parsley and a teaspoon of mayonnaise. Serve with sliced tomatoes and a few olives.

Dinner: 50 g (2 oz) pasta topped with a sauce of 200 g (8 oz) canned tomatoes, 75 g (3 oz) chopped, fried bacon or 100 g (4 oz) canned kidney beans and lots of spinach, mushrooms.

Day 25

Breakfast: 2 pieces of sourdough toast spread with 1 teaspoon soft cheese and topped with 40 g (1½ oz) smoked salmon or 20 g (¾ oz) pumpkin seeds.

Lunch: Half a 600 ml (1 pint) carton of any green-vegetable based soup – served with 2–3 oatcakes spread with 1 tablespoon houmous. Serve with a salad of chopped tomato and onion sprinkled with a little balsamic vinegar.

Dinner: Mexican Peppers (see recipe on page 149). Serve with 50 g (2 oz) quinoa and quarter of an avocado mashed with a little coriander and lime.

Alternative: Stir-fry 125 g (4½ oz) chicken breast with chopped red and yellow peppers and a little fajita seasoning. Serve in one wholemeal tortilla wrap with quarter of an avocado, mashed. If you're vegetarian, fry the peppers alone and add 25 g (1 oz) dry-weight quinoa and 100 g (4 oz) kidney or black beans to the wrap instead of chicken.

Day 26

Breakfast: Savoury Muffin (see recipe on page 134) or two slices of granary toast with 1 teaspoon of peanut butter with a piece of fruit.

Lunch: Niçoise-style salad made from 150 g (5 oz) cooked, cooled new potatoes, 100 g (4 oz) of tuna or 200 g (8 oz) chickpeas, 1 boiled egg, chopped tomatoes, 5–6 black olives and cooked, cooled French beans.

Dinner: 125 g (4½ oz) pan-fried lean steak, or 3–4 falafel balls. Serve with 200 g (8 oz) sweet potato cut into wedges and roasted. Add grilled tomatoes and mushrooms.

Day 27

Time for another benefits audit. If you took a photo before you started drinking, this is a great day to check how your skin has changed – it takes 28 days for skin cells to regenerate so you should clearly notice a difference by now. Also, think about your moods. One side effect of drinking I haven't really talked about is anxiety and depression. Many people find that a heavy night out can lead to rumination, sadness and worry (particularly in the middle of the night). Do you feel happier now you're not drinking? Use that mood boost to keep you going.

Breakfast: Two pieces of granary bread spread with a little mayonnaise. Top with 2 slices of well-grilled bacon or an egg fried in a little oil spray, sliced tomatoes and spinach.

Lunch: Salad of kale, tomato, spring onion and beetroot topped with 50 g (2 oz) feta, halloumi or buffalo mozzarella. Add a little vinaigrette.

Dinner: Coconut Chicken Soup with Fresh Peas (see recipe on page 150).

Alternative: 125 g (4 oz) flavoured chicken breast or tofu served with stir-fry vegetables and 50 g (2 oz) basmati rice.

Day 28

Breakfast: Two eggs scrambled with spinach, a little turmeric and some chilli flakes. 1 slice of sourdough bread.

Lunch: Small jacket potato topped with 2 tablespoons prawn mayonnaise, baked beans or coleslaw and a large green salad.

Dinner: Layer 50 g (2 oz) dry-weight cooked quinoa, a large selection of roasted vegetables and 75 g (3 oz) of houmous in a bowl. Top with a sprinkle of fresh parsley.

Day 29

Breakfast: 40 g (1½ oz) porridge oats made with water. Top with 20 g (¾ oz) pumpkin seeds and 1 tablespoon of natural or Greek yoghurt. Add a dash of cinnamon.

Lunch: Open sandwich of one slice of granary or sourdough bread topped with 200 g (8 oz) sardines (fresh or canned in tomato sauce) or half an avocado, mashed. Serve with a salad of rocket, black olives and cucumber tossed in a little olive oil and vinegar dressing.

Dinner: Kleftiko (see recipe on page 152) or nut roast served with 150 g (5 oz) new potatoes, with carrots and peas.

Alternative: 125 g (4½ oz) roast lamb or beef or 70 g (2½ oz) slice of prepared nut roast with 150 g (5 oz) new potatoes with carrots and peas. Add a little horseradish or mint sauce and some gravy.

Day 30

Breakfast: Two slices of granary toast, 200 g (8 oz) low-sugar baked beans, add a sprinkle of chilli.

Lunch: 150 g (5 oz) of cottage cheese sprinkled with a little turmeric and chilli. Serve with 3–4 oatcakes and lots of cherry tomatoes.

Dinner: 125 g (4½ oz) salmon or trout fillet or a portobello mushroom, grilled. Serve with 50 g (2 oz) pasta spirals mixed with 1 tablespoon of pesto. Add broccoli and peas.

Day 31

This is it your last day – but do you really want to drink tomorrow? It surprised me that whenever I got to the end of the month, I didn't want to drink the next day. As much as the idea that at the end of the month I could go out and have a nice cold glass of wine had sustained me for the last 30 off days, it was always a few days, or even weeks, later that I actually gave in. Turned out I enjoyed the benefits of not drinking and the sense of achievement I felt every time I said no as much as I thought I'd enjoy a glass of wine. I still gave in eventually though …

Breakfast: Chia Pudding (see recipe on page 131) or one Chia Pod, served with one sliced banana.

Lunch: Half an avocado topped with 100 g (4 oz) of fresh salmon or 1 boiled egg mixed with a little mayonnaise. Serve with a side salad of spinach, tomato and 5–6 black olives.

Dinner: Pork with Paprika Mushroom Sauce (see recipe on page 153)

Alternative: 125 g (4 oz) pork steaks or chops or 50 g (2 oz) grilled halloumi with sliced mushrooms. Serve with a fist-sized jacket potato and broccoli.

Ready-to-eat Lunches

If you work in an office that doesn't have a fridge, or simply don't want to take lunch to work some days, that's not a problem. Here're a few suitable lunches you'll find on every high street or in any office canteen.

- Any Pret A Manger, M&S, Leon or Subway salad that includes meat, fish, egg or beans and vegetables.
- A bowl of soup with a small wholemeal roll and 1 tablespoon of coleslaw or a side salad.
- A small pack of sushi (under 350 calories if you're watching your weight) – brown rice or quinoa preferably – with a miso soup.
- Small jacket potato (about fist-sized) served with 2 tablespoons of any traditional topping, such as chilli, baked beans, tuna mayonnaise, prawn mayonnaise or coleslaw.
- Any sandwich on granary, sourdough or rye bread – but pick those under 400 calories if you're watching your weight. Serve with baby carrot, cherry tomatoes or celery sticks.
- 2 tablespoons pasta or potato salad served with a ready-cooked fillet of chicken or salmon or a handful of cashews. Half a bag of salad.

Snacks

Sugary treats are out, but try any of the following if you do feel hungry.

- 25 g (1 oz) of any kind of nuts or seeds.
- Handful of olives.
- 1 tablespoon houmous with crudités or cherry tomatoes.
- 2 oatcakes with 1 teaspoon houmous, peanut butter or cottage cheese.
- 125 g (4½ oz) of natural or Greek yoghurt with a piece of fruit or some berries.
- Two pieces of fruit.
- A cup of miso soup.
- 2 squares of good-quality, high-cocoa chocolate.
- 25 g (1 oz) any cheese with 1–2 oatcakes.

Recipes

Breakfasts

Turmeric Latte (serves 1)

Preparation Time: 5 minutes
Cooking time: 5 minutes

For the spice mix

2 tbsp ground turmeric
2 tbsp ground cinnamon
2 tbsp ground ginger

For the drink

1 tsp honey
200 ml (8 fl oz) milk or dairy alternative

1. Mix 2 tablespoons each of ground turmeric, ground cinnamon and ground ginger in a sealed container and shake well.
2. Add 1 teaspoon of the mix to a cup and add a little hot water and the honey, stir to combine into a paste.
3. Warm the milk or alternative in a pan and then pour over the spice mix, stirring well.
4. Store the rest of the spice mix sealed well until you're ready to use again.

Baked Eggs (serves 2)

Preparation time: 10 minutes
Cooking time: 15 minutes

1 tsp olive oil
2 spring onions, chopped
½ red pepper, chopped
½ red chill, finely chopped
200 g (8 oz) can of chopped tomatoes
1 tsp balsamic vinegar
2 medium eggs
1 tbsp flat-leaf parsley, roughly chopped

1. Heat the oil in a frying pan and fry the spring onions, red pepper and chilli for about 5 minutes until they are softened and golden.
2. Add the chopped tomatoes and vinegar and season well. Bring to the boil, then simmer for a couple of minutes until thickened.

3. Make two wells in the middle of the pan and crack an egg in each. Cook until the whites have started to set then cover and continue to cook until the white is completely cooked through.
4. Divide into two plates, sprinkle with parsley and serve with the sourdough.

Overnight Oats (serves two)

Preparation time: 5 minutes
Chilling time: 30 minutes, or more

85 g (3 oz) rolled oats
1 apple, grated
200 ml (8 fl oz) semi-skimmed milk
100 ml (4 fl oz) plain yoghurt
1 tbsp sultanas
½ tsp of ground cinnamon

1. Put all the ingredients into a bowl and mix well. Place in the fridge and chill for at least 30 minutes, ideally overnight.
2. Simply divide in two and serve – if it's a bit too thick for your taste, add a little more milk or some water and stir.

Chia Pudding (serves 2)

Preparation time: 5 minutes
Cooking time: 20 minutes (including soaking time)

50 g (2 oz) chia seeds
120 ml (4¾ fl oz) full-fat or semi-skimmed milk

50–60 g (2–2¼ oz) blueberries
50 g (2 oz) walnuts, crushed
cinnamon to taste

1. Place the chia seeds in a bowl and add the milk. Divide into two bowls, stir and leave to sit for five minutes.
2. Stir again being careful to smooth out any lumps. Leave for a further 15 minutes until the seeds swell.
3. Add the blueberries and walnuts. Sprinkle with cinnamon and serve.

Savoury Muffins (makes 6)

Preparation time: 15 minutes
Cooking time: 30 minutes

1 medium courgette, grated
1 medium carrot, grated
250 g (9 oz) self-raising wholemeal flour
40 g (1½ oz) pecorino cheese, grated
a pinch of salt
½ tsp ground white pepper
175 g (6 oz) low-fat plain yoghurt
50 ml (2 fl oz) semi-skimmed milk
2 medium eggs

1. Preheat the oven to 200°C/400°F/Gas Mark 6.
2. Put the grated courgette and carrot in a large bowl. Add the flour, cheese, salt and pepper and toss roughly to mix everything together.

3. In a separate bowl, beat the yoghurt, milk and eggs. Make a well in the centre of the flour mixture and pour in the yoghurt mixture. Roughly combine all the ingredients together. Don't worry if there are still some floury patches, these will cook out once the muffins are baked.

4. Line a six-cup muffin tin with paper cases or simply grease with butter. Divide the mixture between the muffin cups and bake for 25–30 minutes, until a skewer pushed into the middle comes out clean.

5. Remove from the tin and cool on a wire rack until just warm, then serve. Freeze any unused muffins until needed. Simply wait for them to cool, wrap them in cling film and freeze. Defrost them the night before you need one and pop under the grill to warm.

Lunches

Leek and Potato Soup (serves 4)

Preparation time: 10 minutes
Cooking time: 15 minutes

575 g (1¼ lb) floury potatoes
2–3 garlic cloves
salt and pepper
350 g (12 oz) trimmed leeks
celery salt (optional)
4 tbsp coarsely chopped fresh parsley
4 tbsp extra-virgin olive oil

1. Peel and thinly slice the potatoes and garlic. Place in a pan and add 1.2 litres (2 pints) cold water. Bring to the boil and add salt. Cover and simmer for about 10 minutes until the potatoes are soft.
2. Meanwhile, slice the leeks. Add them to the potatoes and simmer for a further 5 minutes or so.
3. Roughly mash up the potatoes using a potato masher. Correct the seasoning with celery salt (if using) and pepper to taste. Stir in the chopped parsley.

Dinners

Tandoori Chicken with Minted Quinoa (serves 6)

Preparation time: 20 minutes, plus overnight marinating
Cooking time: 20–25 minutes

6 small skinless chicken breast fillets, each about 125 g (4½ oz)
300 ml (½ pint) Greek yoghurt
2 garlic cloves, crushed
2.5 cm (1 inch) piece fresh root ginger, peeled and grated
finely grated rind and juice of half a lemon
2 tsp hot curry paste
1 tsp paprika
½ tsp salt
225 g (8 oz) dry-weight quinoa
4 ripe tomatoes, chopped

1 small red onion, peeled and chopped
lemon wedges and mint, to serve

Dressing

juice of 2 lemons
25 g (1 oz) caster sugar
25 g (1 oz) mint leaves
125 g (4½ oz) cucumber
50 g (2 oz) sultanas
4 tbsp extra-virgin olive oil

1. Cut the chicken breast fillets into 2.5 cm (1 inch) cubes. Put the yoghurt in a large bowl with the garlic, ginger, lemon rind and juice, curry paste, paprika and salt. Add the chicken pieces, toss well to coat and leave to marinate in the fridge overnight.
2. The next day, cook the quinoa as directed. Once cooked, add the tomato and onion.
3. Meanwhile, prepare the dressing. Put the lemon juice and sugar in a pan and heat gently until dissolved. Stir in the remaining ingredients, season to taste then remove from the heat.
4. Preheat the grill. Remove the chicken from the marinade and thread onto 6 metal skewers. Grill for 10–15 minutes, turning frequently, until the chicken is charred on the outside but cooked right through. Leave to cool.
5. Spoon the quinoa onto individual plates and top with the skewers. Garnish with lemon wedges and mint.

Vegetarian alternative: Use firm tofu or Quorn instead of chicken.

Salmon Fishcakes (serves 4)

Preparation time: 20 minutes, plus chilling
Cooking time: 35–40 minutes

350 g (12 oz) salmon
450 g (1 lb) potatoes
salt and pepper
6 rashers streaky bacon, rinds removed
4 spring onions, trimmed
25 g (1 oz) butter
1 tbsp lemon juice
1 tbsp chopped fresh parsley
1 egg, beaten
50 g (2 oz) fresh white breadcrumbs
oil for frying

1. Place the salmon in a pan and add sufficient water to just cover. Bring to the boil, lower heat and poach gently for 15–20 minutes, until the fish flakes.
2. Meanwhile, peel the potatoes, cut into even-sized pieces and cook in boiling salted water until tender. Drain well and mash until smooth.
3. Preheat the grill and grill the bacon until just brown, but not crispy. Chop into small pieces.
4. Drain the fish and flake, discarding any bones and skin. Mix the fish with the mashed potatoes and bacon.

5. Chop the spring onions. Melt the butter in a small pan, add the spring onions and cook until beginning to soften. Add to the fish mixture, with the lemon juice, parsley and seasoning. Add just enough beaten egg to bind the mixture; it must be firm enough to shape.
6. With floured hands, shape the mixture into 8 cakes. Brush with beaten egg and coat in the breadcrumbs. Chill in the refrigerator for 30 minutes.
7. Heat the oil in a frying pan and shallow fry the fish cakes in batches if necessary, for about 5 minutes on each side, until golden and crisp. Drain on kitchen paper, then serve immediately.

Vegetarian alternative: Replace the salmon with 475 g (18 oz) roughly mashed butter beans. Add these at the end of step 2, stirring them in so they don't become too smooth. Omit the bacon.

Spiced Quick-Fried Prawns (serves 4)

Preparation Time: About 20 minutes, plus marinating
Cooking Time: 20 minutes

450 g (1 lb) large raw prawns
2.5 cm (1 inch) piece fresh root ginger
1 tsp turmeric
1–2 tsp hot chilli powder
2 tsp black mustard seeds
5 green cardamoms, crushed
1 garlic clove, crushed

5 g (2 oz) butter or ghee
6 tbsp coconut milk

1. Peel the prawns leaving the tail end attached. Using a small sharp knife, make a shallow slit along the outer curve from the tail to the head end and remove the dark vein. Rinse under cold running water, drain and pat dry with kitchen paper.
2. Peel and grate the ginger and put into a bowl with the turmeric, chilli powder, mustard seeds, cardamoms and garlic. Add the prawns, turn to coat with the spice mixture and leave to marinate for about 20 minutes.
3. Heat the butter or ghee in a frying pan until foaming. Add the prawns and cook very quickly, stirring all the time for 2 minutes. Add the coconut milk and simmer for about 4 minutes until the prawns are pink and opaque.
4. Serve with basmati rice.

Vegetarian alternative: Swap the prawns for tofu.

Bruschetta of Mushrooms on Wilted Spinach (serves 4)

Preparation time: 10 minutes
Cooking time: 30 minutes

450 g (1 lb) assorted mushrooms, such as ceps, oyster, morels, shiitake or chestnut
4 tbsp extra-virgin olive oil
salt and pepper
225 g (8 oz) spinach leaves

2 garlic cloves
1 tsp grated lemon rind
25 g (1 oz) raisins
2 tbsp pine nuts
1 leek, trimmed

Dressing

4 tbsp extra-virgin olive oil
1 tbsp lemon juice

1. Preheat the oven to 220°C/425°F/Gas Mark 7. Trim the mushrooms and wipe them with a damp cloth. Toss the mushrooms in 2 tablespoon of the oil and season well. Place on a large baking tray and roast in the oven for 15–20 minutes until cooked. Keep warm.
2. Meanwhile, place the spinach leaves in a large colander and pour over sufficient boiling water to just wilt the leaves. Drain well and squeeze out any excess water.
3. Crush 1 of the garlic cloves. Heat 1 tablespoon oil in a frying pan, add the crushed garlic, lemon rind, raisins and pine nuts and fry gently for 3–4 minutes. Finally, slice the leek, add to the pan with the spinach and stir over a gentle heat until warmed through.
4. Shake the dressing ingredients together in a screw-top jar until combined and season with salt and pepper to taste.
5. Grill the bread on both sides, rub all over the surface with the remaining halved garlic cloves and drizzle over the remaining oil.

6. Place the bread on the plate, serve the mushrooms and spinach on top and add the rest of the dressing.

Spiced Lamb with Spinach and Potato (serves 4)

Preparation time 5 minutes
Cooking time: 25 minutes

4 boneless leg steaks of lamb, each about 150–175 g (5–6 oz)
juice of 1 lemon
3 garlic cloves, crushed
1 tbsp chilli oil
1 onion
575 g (1¼ lb) small new potatoes
2 tsp mustard seeds
4 tbsp vegetable oil
300 g (10 oz) packet frozen leaf spinach
salt and pepper
1 tsp ground cumin
5 cm (2 inch) piece fresh root ginger
1 ½ tsp turmeric
4 tbsp Greek yoghurt
shredded mint

1. Lay the lamb steaks in a shallow dish and sprinkle with half of the lemon juice. Spread half of the garlic over the meat, then sprinkle a few drops of chilli oil onto both sides of each steak. Rub the garlic, oil and lemon juice well into the meat.
2. Peel and chop the onion. Wash the potatoes and halve any larger ones. Preheat the grill.

3. Put the mustard seeds in a dry heavy-based pan over a medium heat, cover and shake the pan until the popping dies down. Add 3 tablespoons of the oil and the chopped onion. Cook, stirring frequently, over a low heat for 5 minutes. Add the potatoes and remaining garlic. Cook for a further 2 minutes.

4. Add the spinach, remaining lemon juice and 1 teaspoon each of salt and ground cumin. Stir until the spinach thaws, then cover and leave to cook for 15 minutes.

5. Meanwhile, peel and grate the ginger and mix with the turmeric and remaining oil. Stir in the yoghurt. Season with salt and pepper.

6. Line the rack of the grill pan with foil, lay the lamb steaks on top and grill for 5 minutes on one side. Turn and spread the yoghurt mixture over the uncooked side of the meat and return to the grill for 5 minutes.

7. Uncover the vegetables towards the end of the cooking time to allow any excess liquid to evaporate. Just before serving, add the black pepper, and more salt if necessary.

Vegetarian alternative: Omit the lamb from the recipe, and serve the spinach and potato mix on a bed of 50 g (2 oz) basmati rice or quinoa.

Chicken with a Simple Vegetable Stew (serves 2)

Preparation time: 10 minutes
Cooking time: 25 minutes

2 x 125 g (4½ oz) chicken breasts

3 tsp olive oil
zest of 1 lemon
1 rosemary sprig, leaves chopped
250 ml (10 fl oz) hot chicken stock
1 shallot, sliced
½ celeriac, chopped
2 carrots, chopped
4 stems purple sprouting broccoli
salt and pepper

1. Slash the chicken breasts a couple of times. Rub 1 teaspoon of the oil all over each piece of chicken, season then rub in the lemon and rosemary. Heat a non-stick frying pan over a medium heat and fry the chicken for about 5 minutes on one side until golden.
2. Turn the chicken over and cook for 5 minutes on the other side. Add 100 ml (4 fl oz) hot stock to the pan, cover, and continue to cook over a low heat for 15 minutes until cooked all the way through.
3. Meanwhile, heat the remaining teaspoon of olive oil in a pan and sauté the shallot for a minute or two until starting to turn golden. Add the celeriac and carrots, stir to mix everything together and pour in the remaining stock. Cover and simmer for 10 minutes until the celeriac is tender. Add the broccoli for the last 3 minutes of the cooking time.
4. Season and serve, spooning the stock over the veg and the chicken juices over the chicken.

Vegetarian alternative: Omit the chicken, double the vegetables and serve on 50 g (2 oz) dry weight quinoa.

Asian Beef and Noodles (serves 4)

Preparation time: 20 minutes, plus marinating
Cooking time: 15 minutes

300 ml (½ pint) beef stock
4 star anise
600 g (18 oz) lean steak
8 large spring onions, trimmed
225 g (8 oz) broccoli florets
225 g (8 oz) mangetout, trimmed
1 sheet thin Chinese egg noodles

Dressing

4 tbsp hoisin sauce
4 tbsp rice wine vinegar
2 tbsp dark soy sauce
2 tbsp peanut oil
2 tsp sesame oil
4 tsp thin honey
salt and pepper

1. Place the stock in a frying pan with the star anise and bring to the boil. Add the beef and simmer for 10 minutes.
2. Meanwhile, blend all the ingredients for the dressing together, seasoning with salt and pepper to taste.

3. Remove the beef from the poaching liquid and add 30 ml (2 tablespoons) of the liquid to the dressing. Slice the beef, toss with half of the dressing and leave to marinate for 30 minutes.

4. In the meantime, prepare the vegetables. Cut the spring onions into 5 cm (2 inch) lengths. Blanch the vegetables separately in lightly salted, boiling water: allow 2 minutes for the broccoli; 1 minute for mangetout; 1 minute for spring onions. Drain, refresh under cold water and dry on kitchen paper. Toss with the remaining dressing and set aside for 30 minutes.

5. Boil the noodles as directed and serve with the beef and vegetables on top.

Vegetarian alternative: Swap the beef for 2–3 portobello mushrooms cut into large chunks. Start at Step 2

Fish Pie with Turmeric Mash (serves 6)

Preparation time: 25 minutes
Cooking time: 30–35 minutes

For the mash

1 kg (2¼ lb) floury potatoes
1 tsp ground turmeric
1 garlic clove, peeled
75 g (3 oz) butter, melted
150 ml (¼ pint) single cream
150 ml (¼ pint) milk
salt and pepper

For the pie filling

450 g (1 lb) cod fillet or a similar firm white fish
450 ml (¾ pint) milk
½ onion, sliced
1 bay leaf
225 g (8 oz) tomatoes
175 g (6 oz) cooked shelled prawns
175 g (6 oz) cooked shelled mussels
1 tbsp chopped fresh dill
50 g (2 oz) butter
25 g (1 oz) plain flour

1. Preheat the oven to 180°C/350°F/Mark 4. For the mash, peel the potatoes and cut into even-sized chunks. Put them in a pan with enough water to cover, and add the turmeric and garlic. Bring to the boil and simmer, covered, until cooked.
2. Drain the potatoes, retaining the garlic. Add the butter and mash smoothly. Add the cream and milk and beat until light and fluffy. Season with salt and pepper to taste.
3. Meanwhile, lay the cod in an ovenproof dish, pour in the milk and add the onion and bay leaf. Cover and cook in the oven for 20 minutes until the fish is firm. Strain off the milk and reserve.
4. In the meantime, plunge the tomatoes into boiling water for 30 seconds, then refresh in cold water and peel away the skins. Cut into quarters, remove the seeds and roughly chop the flesh.

5. Turn the oven up to 230°C/450°F/Mark 8. Flake the cod into a buttered ovenproof dish. Add the prawns, mussels and tomatoes. Scatter over the dill.

6. Melt 25 g (1 oz) butter in a pan, add the flour and cook for 30 seconds. Stir in the reserved milk, and cook, stirring, until thickened. Season with salt and pepper and pour over the fish.

7. Spoon the mash on top of the fish mixture, covering it completely. Dot with the remaining butter and bake in the oven for 10–15 minutes until nicely browned on top.

Vegetarian alternative: Replace the white fish with cubed Quorn and/or firm tofu and the shellfish with butter beans

Chickpeas with Spinach (serves four)

Preparation time: 5 minutes
Cooking time: 15–20 minutes

425 g (15 oz) can of chickpeas
1–2 tbsp ghee or vegetable oil
1.2 cm (1/2 inch) piece fresh root ginger, chopped
1–2 garlic cloves, crushed
1 tsp ground coriander
½ tsp ground cumin
1 tsp paprika
2 tomatoes, finely chopped
Small handful of fresh coriander, roughly torn
225 g (8 oz) spinach leaves, chopped
Black pepper

1. Drain the chickpeas and rinse under cold running water.
2. Heat the ghee or oil in a large heavy-based pan. Add the ginger, garlic and spices and cook for 2 minutes, stirring all the time. Add the chickpeas and stir to coat in the spice mixture.
3. Add the tomatoes, torn coriander and spinach. Cook for 2 minutes, then cover with a lid and simmer gently for 10 minutes. Season with salt and pepper before serving.

Mexican Peppers (serves four)

Preparation time: 15 minutes, plus marinating
Cooking time: 20 minutes

3 onions
2 garlic cloves, crushed
2–3 hot chillies, sliced and deseeded
2 tbsps chopped coriander
grated zest and juice of 2 limes
550 g (1¼ lb) lean steak
6 mixed red, yellow or orange peppers, cut into wedges
1–2 tbsps olive oil
salt and pepper

1. Peel and halve the onions, leaving most of the root end attached so that they will hold their shape during cooking. Cut each half into wedges, working from the root end to the top.
2. Put the garlic, onions, chillies, coriander, lime zest and juice in a shallow dish and mix thoroughly. Cut the steak

into large pieces and add to the dish. Stir well, cover and leave to marinate in a cool place for at least 1 hour – or overnight if possible.

3. Heat the oil in a heavy-based frying pan. Remove the steak and onions from the marinade with a slotted spoon, reserving the marinade. Add the steak and onions to the pan and cook, turning, over a high heat until thoroughly browned on the outside. Remove the steak from the pan.

4. Add the peppers to the pan and cook, turning, over a high heat for about 5 minutes until the onions and peppers are softened

5. Return the steak to the pan, add the marinade, lower the heat and cook for about 5 minutes, stirring occasionally, or until the steak is cooked right through.

Vegetarian alternative: Omit the steak from the recipe and use tofu or mushrooms instead.

Coconut Chicken Soup with Fresh Peas (serves 4)

Preparation time: 30 minutes, plus marinating
Cooking time: 1 hour

225 g (8 oz) skinless chicken breast fillet
3 garlic cloves, 1 crushed and 2 left whole
1 tbsp dark soy sauce
1 tbsp Thai fish sauce
1 tbsp tamarind paste
1 tsp turmeric

2 lemon grass stalks
4 kaffir lime leaves
4 coriander roots, scrubbed
900 ml (1½ pints) chicken stock
6 shallots, peeled
2–4 small red chillies, seeded
2.5 cm (1 inch) piece galangal
2 tbsp sunflower oil
400 g (14 oz) can coconut milk
2 tsp soft brown sugar
125 g (4½ oz) frozen peas
2 tbsp torn coriander to serve

1. Cut the chicken breast across the grain into thin slices; place in a shallow non-reactive dish. Combine the crushed garlic clove, soy sauce, fish sauce, tamarind paste and turmeric. Add to the chicken, toss well, cover and leave to marinate for at least 4 hours.

2. For the soup, roughly chop the lemon grass and lime leaves and place in a mortar with the coriander roots; pound together until well bruised. (Alternatively purée briefly in a food processor). Transfer to a large pan and pour in the chicken stock. Bring to the boil, cover and simmer for 30 minutes. Strain and reserve the stock.

3. Quarter the shallots, chop the garlic cloves and chillies and grate the galangal. Heat the oil in a frying pan, add the shallots, and fry for five minutes. Add to the stock with the coconut milk and sugar. Bring to the boil, cover and simmer for 20 minutes.

4. Stir in the chicken, marinade juices and peas. Return to the boil and simmer uncovered for 5–7 minutes until the chicken is tender.
5. Serve at once topped with coriander.

Vegetarian alternative: Replace the chicken with tofu or chopped aubergine. Use vegetable stock.

Kleftiko (serves 4)

Preparation time: 15 minutes, plus marinating time
Cooking time: 2–2½ hours

8 lamb loin chops, or 4 leg steaks (with bone)
2 lemons
1 tbsp dried oregano
2 tbsp olive oil
2 onions
2 bay leaves
150 ml (¼ pint) dry white wine
150 ml (¼ pint) stock
salt and pepper
lemon wedges, to serve

1. Place the lamb in a single layer in a shallow dish. Squeeze the juice from the lemons into a small bowl or cup and add the oregano, salt and pepper. Sprinkle the mixture over the meat and leave to marinate in a cool place for at least 4 hours, preferably overnight.
2. Preheat the oven to 160°C/325°F/Mark 3. Heat the oil in a large frying pan. Lift the lamb chops out of the marinade and add them to the pan. Cook over a high heat, turning

until well browned on all sides, then transfer to a shallow earthenware casserole.

3. Peel and slice the onions and add to the lamb, together with the bay leaves, wine and stock. Pour in any remaining marinade and season with pepper.
4. Cover the dish with foil. Bake in the oven for 2–2½ hours until the lamb is tender, removing the foil for the last 20 minutes to brown the meat.
5. Before serving, carefully skim off any excess fat. Serve the meat with the juices spooned over with lemon wedges on the side.

Pork with Paprika Mushroom Sauce (serves 4)

Preparation time: 10 minutes
Cooking time 20–25 minutes

15 g (½ oz) dried porcini mushrooms
175 ml (6 fl oz) chicken stock
1 small onion
200 g (7 oz) chestnut or cup mushrooms
2 tbsp vegetable oil
50 g (2 oz) butter
4 pork tenderloin fillets roughly 125 g (4½ oz) each
1 tsp fresh or dried thyme
125 ml (4 fl oz) crème fraîche
1 tbsp paprika

1. Put the porcini mushrooms in a small bowl with 3 tablespoons of the chicken stock and leave to stand. Peel the onion and chop finely. Slice the fresh mushrooms.

2. Heat the oil and 25 g (1 oz) of the butter in a frying pan. Add the pork and cook for about 5 minutes each side. Lift out the pork with a slotted spoon and transfer to a warmed dish; cover and keep warm.
3. Add the onion and thyme to the pan and fry over a gentle heat, stirring frequently, for 5 minutes. Add the remaining butter, then add the fresh mushrooms and cook, stirring, over a moderate heat for 5 minutes.
4. Add the porcini with their soaking liquid and cook for 1 minute, then add the crème fraîche. Stir in sufficient stock to thin the sauce to the desired consistency, then add the paprika. Cook for 2 minutes then check the seasoning. Pour the sauce over the pork to serve.

Vegetarian alternative: Replace the pork with half roasted butternut squash topped with the sauce and serve on a bed of 50 g (2 oz) quinoa.

Juices

If you've got a bit more time to spend mixing up a drink, juices and mocktails can help keep your tastebuds interested all month. Here're some ideas to try …

Kale and Hearty

Get your green juice on with this mix of fruit and green vegetables.

2 handfuls of kale leaves
½ cucumber, peeled and chopped
2 celery stalks
3 apples
2.5 cm (1 in) piece of fresh root ginger

1. Roll the kale leaves into a tight ball before juicing to ensure maximum juice yield.
2. Juice all the ingredients and mix well before drinking.

Berry Treat

Packed with nutrients this tall drink is as healthy as it is tasty.

1 handful of cherries
1 handful of strawberries, tops removed
1 handful of raspberries
1 handful of blueberries
150 ml (6 fl oz) soda water

1. Remove the stones from the cherries.
2. Juice all the ingredients.
3. Pour into a glass filled with ice cubes and mix well.
4. Top with the soda water.

Ruby Anyday

Soft drinks can be sweet – the tartness of the redcurrants in this blend adds a refreshingly sour twist.

2 medium carrots, chopped

1 handful of blueberries
1 handful of grapes
1 small handful of redcurrants
1 small knob of fresh ginger

1. Juice all the ingredients and mix well before drinking.

Minty Sunrise

Who needs tequila when you can create colours like these?

2 carrots, chopped
1 orange, peeled
6 grapes
1 small handful of fresh mint, leaves and stalk
25 ml (1 fl oz) grenadine or cranberry juice

1. Juice all the ingredients together and mix well.
2. Top with a splash of grenadine or cranberry juice.

Ginger Whizz

Ginger will give every drink some zing.

1 lime, peeled
3 cm (1½ in) piece of fresh root ginger
2 carrots, chopped
¼ cantaloupe melon, skin removed, chopped

1. Peel the lime and ginger then chop all the rest of the ingredients.

2. Juice everything.
3. For a longer drink top with 150 ml (6 fl oz) ginger beer.

Pear Drops

Reminiscent of mulled cider this is a great winter option.

5 ripe pears, chopped
2.5 cm (1 in) piece of fresh root ginger
A large pinch of ground cinnamon

1. Juice the pears and ginger.
2. Put the juice into a small pan and sprinkle in the ground cinnamon.
3. Heat very gently and drink while still warm.

Raspberry Delight

This creamy blend from nutritionist Rick Hay makes a brilliant substitute for fruity daiquiris.

1 cup of raspberries fresh or frozen
1 cup of strawberries fresh or frozen
100 ml (4 fl oz) coconut water
100 ml (4 fl oz) coconut milk

1. Juice the raspberries and strawberries.
2. Add the coconut water and coconut milk, mix well.
3. Top with a splash of vanilla essence.
4. Serve with a slice of lemon or lime and top with a splash of vanilla essence.

5. Alternatively make a thicker drink by blending all the ingredients.

Tropical Paradise

Get a turmeric hit with this blend from nutritionist Rick Hay.

½ cup of frozen or fresh mango
½ cup of fresh or frozen pineapple
juice of one lime
1 tsp of turmeric
100 ml of water
100 ml of rice or almond milk
a squirt of agave syrup
fresh mint leaves when ready

1. Add all the ingredients, except the mint, to a blender and whizz until combined. For a frozen style drink add crushed ice instead of water.
2. Serve in a tall glass with a mint garnish.

Mocktails

Lime Rickey

If you're missing mojitos this refreshing lime mix from the team at Drinkaware.co.uk is your answer.

30 ml (2 tablespoons) fresh lime juice

30 ml (2 tablespoons) sugar syrup
15 ml (1 tablespoon) bitters
125 ml (4 fl oz) soda water

1. Put the lime, sugar syrup and bitters into a cocktail shaker with ice and shake.
2. Pour through a filter into a tall glass also filled with ice.
3. Add the soda water and serve with a slice of lime

Virgin Mary

A vodka-free version of the spicy classic from the team at Drinkaware.co.uk.

½ lemon, squeezed
Tabasco
Worcestershire Sauce
4 basil leaves, torn
175 ml (7 fl oz) tomato juice
celery sticks to garnish

1. Squeeze the lemon into a cocktail shaker. Add a dash of Tabasco and a splash of Worcestershire Sauce.
2. Tear the basil leaves and add to the mix. Now add ice and the tomato juice
3. Close the shaker, shake. Taste and add more Tabasco or Worcestershire Sauce if needed. Once you're happy with the taste pour through a strainer into a glass full of ice.
4. Add a celery stick to serve.

Pom Collins

The non-alcoholic version of the Tom Collins was created by the team at Drinkaware.co.uk.

1 slice of lime
60 ml (2¼ fl oz) pomegranate juice
30 ml (1¼ fl oz) soda water
Ice

1. Squeeze the lime slice into a glass. Add ice.
2. Fill with the pomegranate juice, top with soda water, stir and serve.

Bitter Orange

Fans of bitter drinks like Campari should try this creation from the mixologists working at the bar chain Be At One.

60 ml (2 ¼ fl oz) grapefruit juice
15 ml (1 tbsp) lemon juice
1–2 tsp bitter orange marmalade
ginger beer to fill

1. Add the grapefruit juice, lemon juice and marmalade to a cocktail shaker and stir to loosen the jam.
2. Add ice cubes and shake vigorously.
3. Strain into a glass and fill with cubed ice.
4. Fill to the top of your glass with ginger beer.
5. Stir once with a straw and serve.

Java Juice

Coffee isn't just for mornings – try this energy shot from the mixologists at bar chain Be At One.

30 ml (2 tbsp) espresso coffee
30 ml (2 tbsp) palm sugar syrup
200 ml (8 fl oz) coconut water to fill

1. Add all the ingredients and ice cubes into a shaker.
2. Shake vigorously.
3. Strain into a tall glass and serve.

English Country Garden

Missing your mojito? The mixologists at Be at One have come up with this minty alternative.

8 mint leaves
30 ml (2 tbsp) cucumber syrup
23 ml (2/3 tbsp) lime juice
soda water to fill
mint sprig to garnish

1. In a tall glass, muddle the mint.
2. Add ice, cucumber syrup and lime juice and mix with a long spoon.
3. Top with soda water.
4. Garnish with a sprig of mint.

Pina No-Lada

The taste of holidays – without the rum.

100 ml (4 fl oz) coconut water
75 ml (3 fl oz) pineapple juice
25 ml (1 fl oz) coconut cream

1. Pour the coconut water and pineapple juice into a tall glass filled with ice cubes.
2. Add the coconut cream on top.
3. Garnish with a pineapple wedge.

Mint Magic

You'll be swept away to the Deep South with this recipe.

8 sweet mint leaves
150 ml (6 fl oz) lemonade
30 ml (2 tbsp) lemon juice

1. Put the mint in a tall glass and muddle to release the flavour.
2. Add ice cubes and top with the lemonade and lemon juice.
3. Stir with a long spoon and serve with a spiral of lemon peel.

Apple Spritz

A perfect alternative to a white wine spritzer.

25 ml (1 fl oz) elderflower cordial

200 ml (1 fl oz) apple juice
1 kaffir lime leaf or a small handful of mint
150 ml (6 fl oz) sparkling water or soda

1. Mix the cordial with the apple juice.
2. Add the kaffir or mint leaves, stir well.
3. Add ice.
4. Top with sparkling water.

CHAPTER SEVEN

Back to Reality

So that's it, your month is over – you've saved money, avoided hangovers, improved your health and perhaps lost a few pounds but now it's time to return to real life – and real drinking. At this point what happens next is very similar to what happens when you come off a diet – if you simply go back to what you were doing in the first place you'll rapidly be back where you started. That's why one of the primary points of abstinence months is to help break the unconscious and unhealthy habits of drinking, allowing you to form a new relationship with booze that sees you drinking sensibly from now on.

The first step in this is to know what you're aiming for and for most of us that means drinking at a level that doesn't negatively affect health. In the UK, this is defined as drinking no more than 14 units of alcohol a week, spread out throughout the week with at least two alcohol-free days somewhere in between.

The important point here though is that one unit of alcohol is not necessarily one bottle or one glass. An alcohol unit in the UK is classed as 8 g or 10 ml of pure alcohol by volume – as such, the more alcohol a drink contains the smaller the measure that contains 1 unit. This means that one unit is classed as:

- Half a pint (284 ml) of normal strength – 3–4 per cent alcohol – beer, lager or cider
- 25 ml of spirits like gin, vodka or whiskey
- 85 ml of 12 per cent alcohol wine

If you are drinking larger measures than the above or you're drinking a stronger lager or wine (some beers can be closer to 5–6 per cent and many wines are now 13–14 per cent ABV) there's going to be more than one unit in the above measures, let alone if you consume more. Thankfully, there's a handy calculation you can do to work out exactly how much you are drinking:

To work out exactly how many units you are consuming, multiply the amount of fluid you are drinking by its ABV (marked on the bottle as a percentage) and divide by 1,000.

So, say for example, you're drinking a large 250 ml pub measure of 14 per cent Merlot. Multiply 250 by 14 then divide by 1,000 – this gives you 3.5 units in that one glass. As you can see, that's quite a lot. More than four large glasses a week and you're over safe drinking limits – even a small glass of a strong wine contains 1.7 units of alcohol. Other higher-unit examples that might trip you up are: bottled lagers – at 330 ml a serving they often contain 1.3 units per bottle; spirits – many pubs now offer 35 ml as a standard measure of these which is classed as 1.4 units; and then there are pints of premium lagers that usually contain around 5 per cent ABV. One of these will be 3 units – around a fifth of your weekly limit in just one pint.

As a general rule, to stick to the weekly safe limits, you can consume the following ...

- Six pints of normal-strength lager
- Fourteen single measures of spirits – or ten 35 ml pub measures
- One and a half bottles of 12 per cent wine
- Ten bottles of 4 per cent lager
- Just under five pints of strong lager

Why Suggest Any Alcohol At All?

Surely it would be easier to just say that alcohol is bad and that we should all be teetotal instead of trying to get us to stick to the moderate intake that so many of us actively exceed. Actually no, as avoiding alcohol entirely is not necessarily better for us than consuming it at a safe dose – and while this is not a reason for anyone who doesn't drink alcohol to start imbibing, in small doses alcohol actually has a lot of positive effects on the body. Like these:

- US researchers have found that older people drinking moderately perform better on memory tests than teetotallers. It's believed the small amounts of alcohol help preserve levels of proteins that protect part of the brain called the hippocampus involved in memory[71]. Numerous other studies have also shown that moderate drinkers have lower rates of age-related mental decline.

- Alcohol has a protective effect on the heart. It increases levels of HDL cholesterol – the so-called good type of cholesterol that helps lower the more harmful LDL form. It also helps thin the blood, decreasing risk of clots that lead to heart attack and stroke. According to work from the Norwegian University of Science and Technology drinking 3–5 units a week reduces heart-failure risk by 33 per cent[72].

- Type 2 diabetes risk is also lower in moderate drinkers. In fact, consuming a couple of alcoholic drinks a day was estimated to reduce risk by around 30 per cent[73]. Exactly why isn't known but it's believed alcohol consumed with food might slow the speed at which sugar enters the blood which may lower diabetes risk.

- Drinkers' bones are stronger. Women drinking 1–2 alcoholic drinks a day had a lower risk of osteoporosis in a study by the US's Oregon State University[74]. When the researchers took blood samples they found that the level of bone turnover decreased when women were drinking and increased when they weren't and the faster bone turns over, the thinner your bones become.

- Drinkers are generally healthier. A study by French scientists on almost 150,000 drinkers[75] found those consuming between 1–3 drinks a day had lower rates of heart disease, stress and depression and had a lower body mass index, meaning they were also at a healthy weight. Female drinkers also had lower blood pressure.

All of this occurs for a variety of reasons. A little alcohol thins the blood, which might play a role in good heart health. It also lowers stress which impacts on mood, blood pressure and weight. On top of this, beer and wine contain antioxidants which help counteract cellular damage in the body and red wine, particularly, is a good source of resveratrol, a flavonoid believed to be linked to slower aging and better brain health. It's also suggested that the social interaction that occurs when we drink with others also plays an important role in alcohol's health benefits – although with your new found sober-socialising skills this is one benefit you can now achieve without alcohol! The caveat of course is that all of these benefits come not from heavy drinking but moderate consumption, which is why what you're aiming to be from now on is Sensible!

So How Do You Drink Sensibly?

Just as quitting completely was a learning curve and saw you planning, plotting and adjusting your behaviour to make different choices, so is drinking sensibly and having a few tactics in place can make it considerably easier to achieve.

The first tip is to not fall into your old alcohol-based lifestyle – if you've started to fill your life with activities that don't revolve around alcohol, started an early morning exercise regime and begun spending more time with friends who don't drink say, then don't drop all of those things now your sober month is over. The less time you spend in activities that revolve around drinking the easier it will be to achieve the goal of having at least two alcohol free days a week.

The next step is to decide how you want to divvy up those 14 units you are allowed in a week as No, you can't have them all at once. To give you some guidance, hangovers tend to kick in after three units of alcohol, four units is when experts say alcohol starts to impede judgement or behaviour in ways that might get you into trouble, while six units for women and eight for men consumed in one session is classed as binge drinking – and that's never a good idea.

Once you've set your limit, it will help to determine if you're a starter or a stopper. These aren't medical phrases, but more an observation that the world of drinkers is divided into two types of people – those that have no problem having one or two drinks then stopping and switching to soft drinks and those that find that if they start drinking alcohol it's very hard to stop. Knowing which you are can help determine the tactics you should use to limit alcohol on a night out. Stoppers should decide on a number of drinks they're going to have and then either swap to soft drinks when they reach it – or alternate soft drinks in between to stretch their alcohol intake throughout the night. Starters, though, need the opposite approach, starting on soft drinks and switching to alcohol later in the night. As a starter myself I can also tell you it really helps when you do buy that first alcoholic drink to get a soda at the same time – you'll drink that too and get at least a bit more booze-free time under your belt.

Stealth Tactics

The above are all conscious choices that help you cut back, but you can also use some more stealthy tactics to reduce how much you're consuming. The simplest of these is to swap to lower-alcohol versions of the drinks you normally consume. There are now wines out there, for example, that are made from grapes picked earlier in the season before they get too sugary. This limits the alcohol the fruits produce and so these wines only have 8–9 per cent alcohol per volume. You can therefore drink 125 ml of these and still only have one unit (compared with just 85 ml if you're drinking a 12 per cent wine). If you swap from a 5 per cent lager to one of the light brands that contain just 2.9 per cent ABV you can consume one and a half more pints a week (eight and a half in total) and still be within those healthy guidelines. One top tip when consuming low or reduced-alcohol drinks, though, is to drink them extremely cold – they can be sweeter than normal and a bit sickly if they get warm.

Dilution is also your friend. Some might see watering down your drinks as a form of sacrilege, but it's my saviour in life, allowing me to sit for hours over dinner or in the pub and not wake up with a hangover. The obvious examples of dilute drinks in the UK are the white wine spritzer, where soda is added to wine or shandy where lager is topped up with lemonade. Personally my dilution of choice is ice which can make a glass of white or rosé wine last twice as long as it gradually melts – but these are by no means the only examples around the world …

In Germany beer is often combined shandy-style with orangeade, cola or lemon-flavoured sodas or given a dash of sweetness with a splash of fruit juice (cherry is particularly good).

In Singapore you can order a Kip-Lin, which is a mix of beer and tonic water.

In Croatia you'll find a drink called Bambus, which is basically red wine topped up with cola – I was instantly a fan, much to the disgust of the wine-buff publican of my local when I asked for it when I returned. It's also common in Argentina, Chile, South Africa and Spain.

In Australia, the non-drinkers 'alcohol' of choice is the LLB – the lemon, lime and bitters. A mix of lemonade, fresh lime and Angostura bitters, it's a regular Monday night tipple. Technically bitters are alcohol but as only a splash is included, the mixture is pretty much alcohol-free. For a lower-calorie alternative also try soda, lime and bitters.

One thing to be careful of if you are diluting drinks though is diet mixers – they speed up how fast alcohol leaves your stomach and may make you drunker quicker[76]. If you're watching the calories, try mixing with soda or at least pace yourself by putting your glass down between drinks. This is particularly important when you first drink again after your month off, which will have lowered your tolerance to alcohol. While you might have been able to down five pints a night, remain feeling sober then bounce out of bed the next morning bright eyed and bushy tailed, during the month of abstinence some changes will have occurred in your brain. The receptors that get pleasure from alcohol have been reset and levels of enzymes that metabolise alcohol will also have fallen – this combination means you need less alcohol now to feel the effects than you did before. Bear that in mind if you're going out.

Also avoid mixing anything with an energy drink – the high levels of caffeine they contain actually cause a reaction that trigger us to crave more alcohol say researchers at the US's Northern Kentucky University[77]. And anything that makes you crave booze is not helpful for encouraging sensible drinking.

Weights and Measures

If you're in a pub it's relatively easy to gauge how much you're consuming as they supply set measures, but if you're drinking at home where you pour your own measures, or are drinking in a restaurant with bottles of wine on the table it can be a bit more difficult to monitor things. In fact, in a study carried out by the UK Government's Know Your Limits campaign, people asked to pour a standard 25 ml measure of spirits actually served, on average, 38 ml. When asked to pour a unit of wine the average poured was 186 ml, not the 125 ml it should be[78]. If you're serious about cutting back at home, learn to pour accurately. Smaller glasses help here. If you're a spirits drinker, a spirits measure can ensure you're pouring a single not a double and you can buy these on websites like amazon.co.uk or drinkaware.co.uk. If you drink fizzy wines, also invest in a bottle stopper – if you know the wine will keep, it'll be easier to not just finish the bottle for the sake of not wasting it.

When shopping for glasses, don't be tempted by coloured ones – we actually drink faster and pour nearly 10 per cent more into a glass in which we can't clearly see the liquid[79]. We also drink faster from glasses with rounded sides. In a study carried out at the University of Bristol drinkers drink 60 per cent faster from a 'fluted' beer glass than a straight-sided one[80]. Researchers suspect we find it harder to judge the volume in a rounded glass, which makes it harder to measure what we're consuming and how quickly so we overindulge.

If you're drinking from a bottle of wine it can also help to institute a 'no top ups till empty' rule where you wait until your glass is empty before you refill it. This makes it easier to keep track of how many glasses you're consuming – you get added sensible points if you don't top up immediately and fill your glass with water instead and drink that between alcoholic drinks. When you do eventually pour, ensure your glass is fixed firmly on the table and not held in your hand. According to US researchers we pour 12 per cent smaller measures when a glass is on the table than if it's being held[81].

The Perfect Combination

Wherever you're drinking it's also a good idea to adopt a policy of mostly consuming alcohol with food. Having food in your stomach slows the rate at which alcohol enters the bloodstream – in fact the level of alcohol in your blood is roughly half the amount if you drink on a full stomach compared to an empty one. This helps reduce its intoxicating effects making it more likely that you'll keep making sensible choices. Drinking mostly with food may also boost the health promoting effects of alcohol – in a study from Finland's Universities of Helsinki and Tampere, people who had a glass of wine with meals scored highly on measures of physical and mental health – but those who drank their alcohol away from the dinner table didn't get the same boost[82].

For an added bonus, adopt a Mediterranean-style diet. One of the few conditions where there seems to be no safe intake of alcohol is breast cancer – even just one alcoholic drink a day raises a woman's risk – but, elements of the Mediterranean diet including olive oil and the folate found in dark leafy green vegetables may counteract some of this increased risk say Spanish researchers[83]. The principles of the Mediterranean plan are simple – consume lots of vegetables and a moderate amount of fruit, eat fish more than meat, choose carbohydrates in the form of pulses and wholegrains rather than refined, sugary starches and add liberal doses of healthy fats like those found in olives, olive oil and avocadoes. If that sounds familiar it's because it's also extremely similar to the Craving-Busting Diet Plan you'll find in Chapter Six!

Keeping Focused

No one's perfect though – you will overdo it sometimes. Once or twice doesn't matter – but if you find yourself regularly slipping back into drinking too much, then try reusing some of the habit-stopping techniques from Chapter Three (see page 52) to get yourself back on track. Remember, you need to make drinking alcohol a choice you consciously make not a habit you fall back into.

So that's it, you're now well on your way to a life of being a sensible drinker, which frees up some extra willpower and determination to make some other positive changes in your life. Perhaps you want to lose weight, eat more healthily, start exercise, quit smoking or save money – well now is the best time to start, and I'll explain why and give some tips to boost your success in the chapter that follows.

CHAPTER EIGHT

The 360°-Change Plan

When you make a success of a goal like giving up alcohol, something changes within you – not just all those health benefits I talked about in Chapter One, but also how you feel about yourself and your ability to stick with and achieve further goals. That makes right now a great time to also consider changing other elements about your life. Maybe you've always wanted to eat better, start exercising or save some cash, well now is the perfect time to give it a try.

The reason is that success begets success when it comes to making change, do one thing and you become more confident in your ability to achieve a second. When you successfully complete a challenge you raise something psychologists call your sense of self-efficacy and when it comes to making changes, this is like the super-power for getting things done.

Well, those are my words anyway – psychologists would say that self-efficacy is the confidence in your ability to do what's needed to make a change or help you reach a goal in life. That goal could be running a marathon, eating a piece of fruit a day, running your own business within the next year – whatever it is, if your self-efficacy in regards to achieving it is high, you'll be more likely to make it happen.

There are a few reasons why. Firstly, when self-efficacy is high you're more likely to see obstacles that get in your way as hurdles to hop over rather than huge barriers designed to stop your success. At least that's what researchers at Michigan State University found when they studied women losing weight after pregnancy. The number one thing that determined who succeeded and who didn't was not the diet a woman picked but being in the possession of what the researchers called an 'I can' mentality before they started[84]. The women who had this weren't floored by setbacks they encountered; they simply found solutions and got on with things.

When self-efficacy is high you also develop a greater interest in what you're trying to achieve. You might read more on a subject or ask the advice of others on how to make things work – and the more knowledge you have about something the more successful you're likely to be at doing it. People who believe something is going to be a success are also likely to put more effort into achieving their aims – you won't mind spending time after work on a business plan or putting in those miles to train for a marathon if you know it's going to go well, but you might be less inclined if deep down you have your doubts.

So, how do you build your self-efficacy? Well, first think of it as something that strengthens in layers not chunks. Every time you achieve something in life – related to your aim or not – your self-efficacy gets a little bit stronger. Reinforce this by celebrating your successes; every night before you go to bed think of as many things you achieved that day as you can and celebrate them. Remember, the key point is layers not chunks so it doesn't matter how small those achievements are – maybe you simply swapped your normal afternoon chocolate bar for a banana or went for a walk after dinner rather than immediately flumping in front of the TV, that's a win – celebrate it. The more you alert your subconscious to these small achievements the more it'll help build your belief that you can take on greater challenges.

Next, find some role models – and ideally pick people to whom you can relate in some way. When we see people with whom we identify – who look like us, come from the same circumstances as us or face the same daily hurdles as us – achieving something, then we are more likely to believe we can do it too. Read books about celebrities or business people you admire, think about friends, relatives or colleagues who've achieved what you want to do, follow people who inspire you on social media or join mentoring or support groups to find others who are doing well. Learn as much from them as you can.

As well as outside influences, self-efficacy also gets built from within and to action this, you need to let your mind know what you want as our brain's main aim in life is to help us succeed. Focusing on a goal, telling your brain what you want turns on part of the brain called the Reticular Activating System (RAS). The day-to-day job of the RAS is to determine which of the millions of images around us we actually pay attention to. Set a goal to lose weight, for example, let your brain know it's your heart's desire and strangely you'll start to spot some amazing-looking healthy eating recipes in a magazine you're reading or notice a new diet book out that sounds perfect for you. Decide to exercise and you might notice how many people are out for walks in your neighbourhood, which may encourage you to join them. Make a decision to start a blog and you'll see an SEO course at your local leisure centre. All of these things were there before, your brain just didn't bring them to your attention as it thought you wouldn't be interested, but now it knows you want to achieve something related to them it's actively pointing them out. To switch on the RAS, repeat your goal to yourself daily or even better write it down stating clearly and precisely what you want to do. As you do this only use positive phrases – the mind doesn't understand negative words like 'don't', tell it that you 'don't want to smoke' and it just sees the word smoke. Say you want to 'stop eating rubbish' and it sees 'eat rubbish'. Couch your goal in positive phrases like 'I will be a non-smoker' or 'I will eat five portions of fruit and vegetables a day' and it'll move mountains to make that happen.

The tips above will strengthen your general self-efficacy and maximise your ability to achieve any goal, but, just as having some specific advice helped you succeed during your month off alcohol, it can also help with some other common goals.

If You Want to Lose Weight

It's often said that diets don't work, but that's actually not true. They work – if you find one you can stick to and have a plan as to how you're going to keep the weight off when you reach your desired goal. The first step in this is finding the plan that works for you and to do that, it has to include foods you like, fit the lifestyle you lead and suit your body type or you either won't be able to sustain it or it won't get results. If you've dieted a few times, you probably have an idea of what works for you and what doesn't but if you haven't then ask yourself the following questions to get some better ideas.

- How fast do you want to lose the weight? If the answer is quickly, a low-carb, high-protein or low-carb, high-fat plan or a very low-calorie plan is going to work better than something more balanced and moderate.
- How strict do you want to be? If the answer is, not very – a plan using fasting techniques like the 5:2 Diet where you only actively cut calories two days a week might be good for you.
- How fiddly do you want it? Calorie, or other counting plans, are great if you don't mind keeping track of things; if you prefer fewer rules pick plans like intermittent fasting that see you just eating healthily, but restrict how often to get results.
- Do you eat meat? If not, high-fat low-carb, high-protein low-carb or Paleo plans are not going to work well. You'll be better off on a low-fat or calorie-counted plan.
- Where do you carry your weight? If the answer is mostly round your middle and/or you feel sleepy after meals, lower carbohydrate diets might work better for you.

- Do you need others to help? If so, trying one of the big slimming clubs could be key to your success.

Once you've chosen the right plan for you, it's important to go into it in a positive frame of mind. Diets tend to focus on deprivation, but according to the US's Baylor University, focusing instead on what you *can* eat gives better results[85]. So whatever plan you've decided upon spend 10–15 minutes writing a list of every single food you can think of that you can enjoy while sticking to your plan and if you start to feel deprived check this over to find some new ideas.

Just as you did when you were quitting alcohol, always remember one slip up won't trigger you to gain everything you've lost, however, following that one slip up with three days of overeating because you feel guilty or because you've decided to start again on Monday will have negative effects. If you slip up, get started again at your very next meal.

Finally, while you're on whatever eating regime you've chosen, start thinking about how you're going to keep this weight off. The very act of losing weight means you can't eat as much as before and maintain the same weight. If you simply go back to eating the way you were before, the weight will just go back on. Think about what habits you need to break and what steps can you take now to change your behaviour. All the tips you learnt in Chapter Three on breaking the habit of alcohol (see page 52) also work on changing eating habits too so go back and use those. Also, get exercising – contrary to what many think, it's not a great way to lose weight as it's a lot faster to eat calories than burn them, but it's brilliant at helping you maintain it. Ninety per cent of the people questioned by the National Weight Registry (who follow people who've successfully lost and kept off a lot of weight), do an hour of some kind of exercise every day to help themselves stay slim[86]. If you're not a fan of exercise, the tips on page 188 can help change that.

If You Want to Eat More Healthily

The first step in doing this is to determine exactly what this means to you – healthy eating is a very nebulous term and even experts fight about what it means – should we simply be banning processed foods, eating mostly plants, quitting grains our grandparents didn't eat or just cooking properly from scratch? Nebulous goals are hard to meet, so your first step in becoming a healthier eater is to decide exactly what you want to achieve. Is it simply eating five portions of fruit and vegetables every day; cutting back on sugar and salt; banning unprocessed foods or cooking more? Determine exactly what change or changes you're going to make and write those goals down.

Now look at how you can make them happen. If it's starting to do something new like adding more fruit and vegetables to your day, one of the most successful techniques you can use is called anchoring. This is where you anchor the behaviour to something you already do – so, if you want to eat more fruit and vegetables, for example, tell yourself you'll have a banana on the bus to work every morning and that each day at lunch you'll add a portion of vegetables as a side dish. Do that and you'll soon make eating the healthy food a part of your normal behaviour and the habit will stick.

If you're trying to break a habit like reaching for takeout when you come home tired, the absolute best tactic you can use is the If–Then approach that you've already learnt (see page 55). Think of all the situations in which you might act in ways that will counteract your eating goal and come up with If–Then solutions for them. For example …

- If I come home late and want a takeaway – then I will ensure there's always a healthy meal in the freezer I can warm up quickly in the microwave.
- If I tend to serve myself too large portions – then I will serve my food on a smaller plate and wait 30 minutes after finishing before I eat anything else.
- If I go out for lunch with friends from work – then I will order a starter and a salad to make sure I get my vegetables in.

Finally, start calling yourself a healthy eater. As soon as you start calling yourself something, you're more likely to become it as your brain starts to see the name as part of your identity and it will start to seek out behaviour to reinforce it says research from the US's Winona University[87].

If You Want to Quit Smoking

Fewer people than ever are now smoking in the UK. A combination of higher cigarette prices, smoking bans in pubs and more effective quitting methods mean that only 19 per cent of the population now smoke[88]. Here's some advice to help you join the quitters.

The reason smoking is arguably the hardest of all the bad habits to break is that not only do you have to break the habit of smoking; you have to do so while coping with physical withdrawal symptoms. As such, you might find it easier to quit using one of the many smoking cessation aids available.

The first type of these is nicotine replacement therapies (NRTs) like nicotine gum, patches or inhalers. You use these to supply the body with nicotine while you break the habits and associations of smoking, and then in time slowly wean yourself off the nicotine itself. You can buy NRTs from pharmacies, or get them on prescription from your GP.

Instead of NRTs you may prefer to use e-cigarettes. These are designed to give smokers a way to take in nicotine without exposure to the 4,000-odd other chemicals contained in cigarettes that cause the diseases associated with smoking. You can use e-cigs to quit, but many users merely use them to replace normal cigarettes. E-cigarettes are not available on prescription.

If you'd prefer to not use nicotine replacement, you have two options. Firstly, there are two prescription medications that can help you quit. One is called Champix and this works by attaching to nicotine receptors in the brain. This has two effects. It releases a small amount of dopamine which helps reduce feelings of withdrawal and, because the receptors are blocked by the drug, if you do smoke the nicotine doesn't get into them and so you don't feel any pleasure from it. The combination is extremely effective. You take it for twelve weeks, beginning one to two weeks before you decide to quit. The other drug is called Zyban and it's one of the great accidental discoveries of medicine. The drug was developed as an anti-depressant but during trials it was found that people using it to boost mood also found it easier to quit smoking. It's suspected to alter levels of neurotransmitters in the brain that fight withdrawal. Again, you start taking the drug before you officially quit. Both drugs are available on prescription and your GP can talk you through which might be right for you.

Of course it's also completely possible to quit smoking cold turkey – where you just quit and rely on willpower and craving control to break the habit and any withdrawal symptoms. It can be a bit tougher than quitting with the help of a cessation method, but every year thousands of successful quitters do it so if you think it's right for you then go for it.

Once you know how you want to quit, grab a pen and paper – it's time to make the list of reasons why you should so you can refer to it if motivation slides. Again, it's important here to word these correctly so if you didn't do the quiz on page 61 to tell you whether you're motivated by avoiding the harm of smoking or enjoying the benefits you'll get from quitting, do that now. Once you've finished that list, then it's also a good idea to write down some If–Then sentences to help you plan how you're going to handle situations when you might normally smoke – for example, when you're first asked to go out for a smoke break at work, how you'll handle stressful days or what happens when you go out with smoking friends.

As with so many habits you also need to have a plan in place to tackle cravings when you give up smoking. These can be physical or psychological and so it's a good idea to have some tactics in place if they strike. Here are some ideas specifically shown to work for smokers …

- Breathe through a straw. It mimics the action of smoking and can be helpful until the urge passes. Breathe in for five seconds, hold for two, then breath out for five. Repeat for five breaths.
- Sniff black pepper oil. Add three drops of this to a tissue and inhale if you feel a craving coming on. Studies published in the journal Drug and Alcohol Dependence showed this cut craving for nicotine – possibly because the pepper causes a similar feeling at the back of the throat to cigarettes[89].
- Get moving. Researchers in Australia have found that running, cycling and walking all stop cigarette cravings in their tracks – if a craving strikes, get your shoes on and head outside for 10–15 minutes while it passes[90].

Once all of the above is in place, simply set yourself a date to become a non-smoker. Having a clear date in mind is important if you're going to use drugs like Champix or Zyban as it allows you to time taking the medication so it's at full power when you have your last cigarette. For women, it can also help to schedule quitting in the second half of your menstrual cycle. The combination of high progesterone to low oestrogen at this point actually makes breaking habits easier say researchers at the Perelman School of Medicine in Pennsylvania[91]. Setting a date also helps focus your brain on what's going to happen and gets your reticulating activating system on board. The date might be that very day, the next day, or two weeks later, but the main point is that when you reach it, you have no cigarettes in the house and you know what you're going to do to fight cravings or how to handle certain situations. From that moment on, start referring to yourself as a non-smoker – and focus on staying that way.

If You Want to Start Exercising

Health experts say we should be doing 150 minutes of moderate exercise every week to stay healthy but in fact only 67 per cent of men and 55–58 per cent of women get that amount[92]. There are three main reasons why we don't work out or why we quit when we start: we don't get results, we don't enjoy it and we don't think we can find the time. Breaking down the barriers to each of these is the key to making exercise become a habit.

How to get results

All exercise is good exercise, but if you want to get appreciable results from your workout you need to choose the right type of exercise for the goal you're trying to achieve.

Cardiovascular exercise

This works your heart and lungs and includes exercises like running, walking, swimming, cycling, rowing, skating, dancing and classes like step or aerobics. It's excellent for burning calories and so is good if your aim is weight loss. It also strengthens the heart and lungs, builds bones and aids immunity and so is brilliant if your aim is improving all-round health. By boosting circulation, exercise also raises energy, aids sleep and fights fatigue. It's also good for reducing stress.

Strength/toning work

This improves muscle definition and tone – and is good for changing body shape – whether you'd prefer to be bigger, smaller or just more lifted in places. Building lean muscle also revs up the metabolism so you burn more calories even at rest, which makes it also good for weight control or fat loss. Good strength workouts include weight training, CrossFit, toning classes like Body Pump and reformer-based Pilates classes that use high resistance.

Stretching

This includes classes like yoga or Pilates and it improves flexibility and decreases tension in the body. It's good for reducing stress, boosting body image, toning muscles and building all round health and mobility but you don't burn a lot of calories doing it so it's not the best choice if you want to lose weight.

Mindful exercises

These use the body to help still and focus the mind. Yoga, tai chi and chi gung all fit into this category. They're excellent if you want to use exercise to fight stress.

Find a workout you enjoy:

The workout you're going to stick at is one that makes you both healthy and happy. If every time you go out for a run you despise every second of it, you are never going to make it a habit – remember, part of making a habit is that your body needs to feel it's getting some kind of reward from the activity. You will however get that reward if you find a workout you enjoy and to do that, here are some of the questions to ask yourself:

- Do you like to work out alone or with other people?
- Do you want to compete against others or do you dislike the pressure of teams, partners or races?
- Do you want to work out inside or outside?
- Do you find gyms/classes/teams welcoming or intimidating?
- Which sports did you love at school – and can you incorporate those into exercise now?
- What about in your teens and twenties – did you love dancing, rollerblading or gymnastics – and again, can you do that now?
- Do you like intense exercise like boxing or running, or would you prefer something more fun like a dance class or relaxing like yoga or hiking?

Weigh up your answers and make a list of exercises that might fit the bill – get creative when you do this. Many of us have an image of what exercise must be – jogging, cycling, lifting weights – but dancing, rollerblading, rock climbing, skiing, ice skating, sailing a boat, digging in the garden, swimming, hiking, archery, tai chi, badminton and five-a-side football all get you moving and all count as exercise to some degree. Once you've got your list together, give all the workouts on it a try – at least once, ideally twice. The more you try the sooner you'll find something you truly love. When you do a workout, try this exercise. Think about how much you're going to enjoy the workout and mark it out of ten. When you're finished mark it again on how much you really did enjoy it. In studies at the University of British Columbia, almost every one enjoyed a workout more than they thought they would – and this helped boost their intentions to work out again[93].

Make time, don't try and find it:

Decide when you are going to work out, put it in your diary and then stick to it. Some people may need a strict schedule to do this, in which case going to classes or joining a team or a club can give you a routine. If you're more self-motivated, then putting workouts in your diary and sticking to them just as if they were appointments with the doctor or the dentist can often be enough.

One thing that can also help you find time is the latest evidence showing that if you work hard in the gym you can get results from far shorter periods of exercise than you may ever have thought possible. Studies have shown that working out for as little as 20 minutes alternating short bursts of hard exercise with gentler sets of recovery improves fitness just as much as long, slow, steady sessions – and can also help people lose body fat. This is called High Intensity Interval Training (HIIT) and you'll now find numerous gyms offering short sharp workouts based on the idea. If your doctor says it's okay to try HIIT on your own, simply try one of the following speedy workouts:

- Get on an exercise bike and warm up for 3–4 minutes. Now, cycle as fast as you possibly can for 30 seconds. Pedal slowly for four minutes – then repeat. Do this four times.
- Do a short warm up then follow by a circuit of ten burpees, five push-ups, ten star jumps, five squats then ten medicine ball slams. Do as many circuits of this as you can in five minutes, then take a one minute break. Repeat the circuit twice more then cool down.
- Warm up for 3–4 minutes then row as fast as you can for eight seconds, recover completely for 12 seconds. Repeat for 20 minutes.

And also don't forget that exercise doesn't have to be done in the gym – running or cycling to work instead of getting the bus or train counts as a workout and, depending how far away you live, probably takes about the same amount of time (with the added bonus that active commuters tend to arrive at the office happier than those that drive in).

If You'd Like More Money

There're two ways to make money – you can try and earn more of it, or you can plug the gaps in your spending that waste it. The most successful budgeters do a combination of both.

When it comes to saving money, it's a matter of doing the sensible things – pay off loans charging interest as fast as possible, shop around to save money on things like car insurance, ask what luxuries you won't really miss if you get rid of them from your life, buy generic products rather than big name brands and use money-saving deals when possible. What's therefore more exciting to explore is the explosion of ways you can make money, completely legally, outside of your day job.

You see, when we think of making money, many of us focus on trying to increase what we earn from the main way we make our living and yes, while getting a pay rise or a promotion will see more cash in your pocket, it's not something that's necessarily under your control, nor can you rely on it happening regularly. The development of what experts call the sharing economy, however, opens up additional income streams to many of us. Setting things up might only take an hour or two – but it can pay dividends for months or years.

The idea of the sharing economy is that you rent your skills or unused assets (be that a room in your home, a car that sits idly in your driveway or possessions you no longer use) to other individuals. According to a recent report by JP Morgan people can boost their income by up to 15 per cent by expanding their income stream in this way[94]. Here are some ideas worth investigating:

- Do you have a spare room you can rent out using websites like Airbnb? You don't have to do it all the time, even renting just one night a week would net you £2,500 a year if you charged £50 a night.
- Do you have a car parking space you don't use? Let other people park on it. You can earn up to £400 a month via some drivesharing websites especially if your house is near a station, hospital or city centre that has limited parking.
- Are you handy at putting up shelves or even just willing to go to IKEA and pick up the purchases for someone who can't face doing it? Task-sharing sites like Task Rabbit let you volunteer for simple jobs – and you set your own price.
- Love to take photographs? Upload these to amateur photo syndication websites and you could earn £10 every time someone buys them to use on a blog or book cover, or even more if they use it in an advertising campaign.
- Declutter. Online retailer Gumtree estimates that the average person has £1,000 of unwanted goodies around their home. Do a declutter and sell as much as you can. If you get good at online selling you can also offer to sell goods for friends or family who find listing things too time consuming and take a small percentage of what they raise.

To maximise your use of the sharing economy, ask yourself what you can offer other people that they might need. Focus particularly on things you love to do as then it won't feel like taking on another job, instead just making money from something you enjoy – then do a Google search for companies offering that service to people. You'll be amazed at what's out there and, if you have something to offer but can't find a business offering it yet, maybe you've stumbled on the next Airbnb or Uber!

If You Want More Time

A 2013 study by the insurer Direct Line suggested that to be happy we need seven hours of free time to ourselves each day – but with a combination of overtime and other priorities getting in the way, we're falling short by an average of 2 hours and 45 minutes. Now, it's true we're living in a time-poor society but it's also true that we waste a lot of time each day by doing things inefficiently or that we don't want or really need to do. Here's how to free up some extra hours in your day to relax, recharge or do the things you love.

The first thing to do is identify your time personality. We all waste time in different ways and knowing what you do can be the key to snatching back some of those missing minutes. Which one of the following are you?

- Procrastinators have trouble getting started on tasks. You'll spend ages playing around on the Internet or doing menial tasks like filing rather than getting down to what truly needs to be done. If this sounds like you, use a technique called Pomodoro to get started. Break the task into manageable chunks, sit down, set a timer and for 15 minutes just do what you need to do and focus on it completely. Often you'll get the task done completely or have the urge to keep going at least.

- Multitaskers skip from task to task. Contrary to popular belief this does not save time – in fact, it takes our brain a second or two to refocus between tasks – longer if the tasks are more complex – leading some experts to say that multitasking may actually drain 40 per cent of our productive time. Make a priority list each day and work through it one thing at a time.
- People Pleasers spend time doing things that aren't their responsibility or that they don't want to do but feel obliged to. Solving this is easy. Learn to say no more often. Make it a rule that you don't say yes to things because you think you should do them – only say yes to things you want to do or need to do for some clear, constructive reason.
- Under-estimators think things should always take less time than they should. Beat this by assuming everything is going to take 20–40 per cent more time than you think it will and only schedule what can fit in your day.

If you're not actually sure where your time is going, it can help to do a mini-audit: Spend three or four days with a pen and paper constantly by your side. Whenever you start doing something (even if it's just making tea or checking an email) write down the time you started and stopped. At the end of the three days, add up how long you spend doing everything and look for surprises. Common time sappers include checking email too often, spending 15 minutes on a call that should take five and chatting while you're working late instead of focusing solely on the task that needs to be completed. How many are you guilty of? Your time audit can also help you find dead time in your day that you can use to carry out simple tasks. Can you return phone calls while you walk home? Pay bills while you wait for the kettle to boil? Go for a run at lunchtime rather than sitting at your desk mindlessly refreshing Facebook or install an expenses app on your phone that allows you to log your accounts on the train or bus ride home. Think where you have dead time and what might be a better use for it.

When it comes to time management, it's also very helpful to know about Parkinson's Law, the basic premise of which is that tasks expand to the time you give. Setting goals can help here – decide how long you have for a task (being completely realistic) and tell yourself it will be completed by then. Even mark the timing on your daily to-do-list or, for longer-term projects, put the completion date on your calendar. Build in a few breaks in case things run over and to give yourself time to recharge. You'll be amazed at how much more you get done when you set yourself a cut-off point.

Finally, it might also help to spend a little bit of time doing something for others. This might sound odd – after all if you don't think you've got enough hours in the day, why would you want to add another item to your to do list? But according to research at the University of Pennsylvania, when we give up time to help others we feel we have more time to spend on ourselves[95].

If You Want to Digitally Detox

According to the communications watchdog Ofcom, the average person today spends eight hours and 41 minutes staring at some kind of screen – that's 20 minutes longer than we spend asleep. We might think it's a harmless pastime, but actually, experts are saying the constant stimulation of our minds that screens offer is interfering with health and wellbeing, it's messing with our sleep, affecting our attention spans in ways that mean we're becoming more impatient and less tolerant to others and it puts barriers up in our relationships. Not to mention how much time we'd free up if we weren't spending so long watching kittens on the Internet.

Cutting back on screen time is referred to as digital detoxing – and while it seems like it would be easier to quit than some of the other habits we've discussed in this book, that might not be so. Online interaction can actually give us the same buzz as alcohol or smoking as we get a little jolt of dopamine whenever someone replies to our text, comments on our Facebook post, likes our Instagram picture or retweets our tweet. This helps explain the compulsiveness that many people display checking their gadgets throughout the day – they're craving the dopamine hit.

As such, digitally detoxing takes as much planning as quitting smoking, eating less or taking that month off the booze. Here are five steps to try …

1. Set limits. Decide what times of day or during which situations you won't check your gadgets – i.e. never on holiday or never when you're sitting with your partner or children. And don't breach those limits.

2. Employ a blocker. There's a growing amount of technology out there that can help you control your screen time by simply not allowing you to access certain sites at certain times of day. Try Self Control (selfcontrolapp.com) or Rescue Time (rescuetime.com).

3. Retro-post. Yes, it's fun to tell your social media followers when you've done something amazing, but do it after the event not during it. The hashtag latergram was developed for this very purpose and you can use the idea across all social media – engage yourself fully in an event, post when it's over.

4. Strengthen your 'mindfulness' neurons. Your ability to focus is like a muscle, you need to exercise it to build it. So, every day, practise focusing on just one thing, it could just be the view out of the window, for five minutes. After 30 seconds you're going to feel bored, but notice that then let it go. Every time you do that you're strengthening the neural connections that stop you needing constant stimulation.

5. Switch off your screen and go and do something less boring instead. That was the tagline of the popular TV

show *Why Don't You?*, which was on when I was growing up and while that might have been a while back, it's just as relevant now as it was then. When you're mindlessly scrolling through website after website, ask yourself what am I getting from this? If it's laughter, support, knowledge or another positive emotion, continue, but if it's just passing the time, it's time to de-tech, detox and find something better to do.

The End

So there you have it – how to change your life in eight easy chapters. What started as a book you bought just to make the challenge of saying no to a nightly glass of wine for 30 days could end up changing your life, improving your health, altering your shape or at least freeing up a bit more time or cash. I bet you didn't expect that from the title when you picked it up.

I hope that while reading it you've learnt a lot about how the mind works and how habits are formed, and realised that every single one of us has the ability to break habits that are negatively impacting our lives – whether that just be drinking a little bit more than you might like or any of the other elements I've discussed.

And, if you see me down the pub at any point remember that might not necessarily be booze in my glass. But if it is and you're buying I'll have a red wine and cola – with a large glass of ice on the side!

Endnotes

1. British Beer and Pub Association, figures for 2015
2. Samsung 'Time of Our Lives' Report, 2016
3. Mysupermarket.com, 2016
4. Alcohol Concern
5. Dryathlon
6. Alcohol Concern
7. Mysupermarket.com, 2016
8. Macmillan Go Sober for October
9. Alcohol Concern
10. Voucherbox.co.uk, 2015
11. World Health Organisation Global status report on alcohol and health, 2014
12. Drinkaware press release, 2016
13. Public Health England Local Alcohol Profiles for England, 2015
14. Health and Social Care Information Centre (2015) Health Survey For England 2014 Trend Tables
15. Strang J et al. 'Addictions, Dependence and Substance Misuse' in the Annual Report of the Chief Medical Officer 2013: 'Public Mental Health Priorities: investing in the evidence'.
16. 'Our Liver Vacation: Is a Dry January Really Worth It?' *New Scientist*. December 2013
17. Mehta G et al., 'Short Term Abstinence from Alcohol Improves Insulin Resistance and Fatty Liver Phenotype in Moderate Drinkers.' Presented at the AASLD Meeting, San Francisco, 2015

18. Chan JK, Trinder J, Colrain IM and Nicholas CL, 'The Acute Effects of Alcohol on Sleep Electroencephalogram Power Spectra in Late Adolescence.' *Alcohol Clinical and Experimental Research*. February 2015; 39 (2): 291–9

19. Askgaard G, Grønbaek M, Kjaer MS, Tjønneland A and Tolstrup JS. 'Alcohol Drinking Pattern and Risk of Alcoholic Liver Cirrhosis: A Prospective Cohort Study', *Journal of Heptatology*. 2015 May; 62(5): 1061–7

20. Marques-Vidal P et al. 'Different Alcohol Drinking And Blood Pressure Relationships in France and Northern Ireland: The PRIME Study', *Hypertension*. 2001 Dec 1; 38(6): 1361–6

21. Eiler WJ 2nd et al. 'The Apéritif Effect: Alcohol's Effects on the Brain's Response to Food Aromas in Women', *Obesity (Silver Spring)*. 2015 Jul; 23(7): 1386–93

22. Confused.com, 2014

23. Booze Up, 2016

24. Alcohol in the Workplace Factsheet: Institute of Alcohol Studies, 2014

25. Verster JC et al. 'Hangover Research Needs: Proceedings of the 5th Alcohol Hangover Research Group Meeting', *Current Drug Abuse Reviews*. 2013 Sep; 6(3): 245–51

26. Palamar JJ, Acosta P, Ompad DC and Friedman SR, 'A Qualitative Investigation Comparing Psychosocial and Physical Sexual Experiences Related to Alcohol and Marijuana Use among Adults', *Archives of Sexual Behaviour*. 2016 Jul; 20: 1–14

27. Dolder PC et al. 'Alcohol Acutely Enhances Decoding of Positive Emotions and Emotional Concern for Positive Stimuli and Facilitates the Viewing of Sexual Images', *Psychopharmacology (Berl)*. 2016 Sep 19 (e-pub)

28. Custard Online Marketing, 2015

29. De Visser RO, Robinson E and Bond R. 'Voluntary Temporary Abstinence From Alcohol During "Dry January" and Subsequent Alcohol Use', *Health Psychology*. 2016 Mar; 35(3): 281–9.

30. Presented at Obesity Week 2014: The American Society for Metabolic and Bariatric Surgery and the Obesity Society Joint Annual Scientific Meeting; November 2014

31. Patrick VM and Hagtvedt H. '"I Don't" versus "I Can't": When Empowered Refusal Motivates Goal-Directed Behaviour.' *Journal of Consumer Research*. 2012 Aug; 39 (2): 371–381

32. Halonen JI et al: 'Living In Proximity Of A Bar And Risky Alcohol Behaviours: A Longitudinal Study.' *Addiction*. 2013 Feb; 108(2): 320–8

33. Wansink B, Painter JE and Lee YK. 'The Office Candy Dish: Proximity's Influence on Estimated and Actual Consumption'. *International Journal of Obesity* (Lond). 2006 May; 30(5): 871–5

34. Gollwitzer PM, Sheeran P, Michalski V and Seifert AE. 'When Intentions Go Public. Does Social Reality Widen The Intention-Behaviour Gap?' *Psychological Science*. 2009 May; 20(5): 612–18

35. Free C et al. 'Smoking Cessation Support Delivered via Mobile Phone Text Messaging (txt2stop): A Single-Blind Randomised Trial.' *The Lancet*. 2011 Jul; 2:378 (9785): 49–55

36. Hung IW and Labroo AA. 'From Firm Muscles to Firm Willpower: Understanding the Role of Embodied Cognition in Self-Regulation.' *Journal of Consumer Research*. 2011 April; 37(6): 1046–64

37. Brinol P and Petty RE. 'Overt Head Movements and Persuasion: A Self-Validation Analysis.' *Journal of Personality and Social Psychology*. 2003 Jun; 84 (6): 1123–39

38. Knäuper B et al. 'Fruitful Plans: Adding Targeted Mental Imagery to Implementation Intentions Increases Fruit Consumption.' *Psychology & Health*. 2011 Feb; 26 (5): 601–17

39. De Visser RO, Robinson E and Bond R. 'Voluntary Temporary Abstinence from Alcohol During "Dry January" and Subsequent Alcohol Use.' *Health Psychology*. 2016 Mar; 35(3): 281–9

40. Baumeister RF and Tierney J *Willpower: Rediscovering the Greatest Human Strength* (Penguin, 2011)

41. Lally O, Van Jaarsveld CHM, Potts HWW and Wardle J. 'How are Habits Formed: Modelling Habit Formation In The Real World.' *European Journal of Social Psychology*. 2010 Oct; 40 (6): 998–1009

42. Shirran M & M with Graham F *Pause Button Therapy®* (Hay House, 2012)

43. Hallam R, Rachman S and Falkowski W. 'Subjective, Attitudinal and Physiological Effects of Electrical Aversion Therapy.' *Behaviour Research and Therapy*. 1972 Feb; 10(1): 1–13

44. Briñol P, Gascó M, Petty RE and Horcajo J. 'Treating Thoughts As Material Objects Can Increase Or Decrease Their Impact On Evaluation.' *Psychological Science*. 2013 Jan 1; 24(1): 41–7

45. Tam L, Bagozzi RP and Spanjol J 'When Planning is Not Enough: The Self-Regulatory Effect Of Implementation Intentions On Changing Snacking Habits.' *Health Psychology* 2010 May; 29 (3), 284–92

46. 'Stress in America', American Psychological Association 2011

47. Baumeister RF and Tierney J *Willpower: Rediscovering the Greatest Human Strength* (Penguin, 2011)

48. Gailliot MT, Baumeister RF. 'The Physiology of Willpower: Linking Blood Glucose to Self-Control.' *Personality and Social Psychology Review*. 2007 Nov; 11(4): 303–27

49. Milkman KI. 'Unsure What the Future Will Bring? You May Overindulge: Uncertainty Increases the Appeal of Wants Over Shoulds'. *Organizational Behavior and Human Decision Processes*. 2012 Nov; 119 (2): 163–76

50. Webb TL and Sheeran P. 'Can Implementation Intentions Help to Overcome Ego-Depletion?' *Journal of Experimental Social Psychology*. May; 39 (2003): 279–86

51. Inzlicht M, Schmeichel BJ and Macrae CN. 'Why Self-Control Seems (But May Not Be) Limited.' *Trends in Cognitive Sciences*. 2014 March; 18 (3): 127–33

52. Dolcos S and Albarracin D. 'The Inner Speech of Behavioural Regulation: Intentions and Task Performance Strengthen When You Talk to Yourself as a You.' *European Journal of Social Psychology* 2014 Oct; 44 (6): 636–42

53. Muraven M and Slessareva E. 'Mechanisms Of Self-Control Failure: Motivation And Limited Resources.' *Personality and Social Psychology Bulletin* 2003 Jul; 29(7): 894–906

54. Wang J et al. 'Alcohol Elicits Functional and Structural Plasticity Selectively in Dopamine D1 Receptor-Expressing Neurons of the Dorsomedial Striatum.' *Journal of Neuroscience*. 2015 Aug 19; 35(33): 11634–43

55. Knäuper B, Pillay R, Lacaille J, McCollam A and Kelso E. 'Replacing Craving Imagery With Alternative Pleasant Imagery Reduces Craving Intensity.' *Appetite*. 2011 Aug; 57(1): 173–8

56. Krahn L and Gordon IA. In Bed With a Mobile Device: Are the Light Levels Necessarily Too Bright For Sleep Initiation? (Abstract). Presented at *SLEEP*, 2013

57. Haralabidis AS et al. 'Acute Effects of Night-Time Noise Exposure on Blood Pressure in Populations Living Near Airports.' *European Heart Journal*. 2008 Mar; 29(5): 658–64

58. Kräuchi K, Cajochen C, Werth E and Wirz-Justice A. 'Warm Feet Promote the Rapid Onset of Sleep.' *Nature*. 1999 Sep 2; 401(6748): 36–7

59. Buscemi N et al. 'The Efficacy and Safety of Drug Treatments for Chronic Insomnia In Adults: A Meta-Analysis of RCTs.' *Journal of General Internal Medicine*. 2007 Sep; 22(9): 1335–50

60. Lui A et al. 'Tart Cherry Juice Increases Sleep Time in Older Adults with Insomnia.' *The FASEB Journal* 2014, April; 28 (1) (830.9)

61. Winograd RP, Steinley D and Sher K. 'Searching for Mr. Hyde: A Five-Factor Approach to Characterizing "Types Of Drunks".' *Addiction Research and Theory*. 2016; 24(1): 1–8

62. Bègue L, Bushman BJ, Zerhouni O, Subra B and Ourabah M. '"Beauty is in the Eye of the Beer Holder": People Who Think They are Drunk Also Think They are Attractive'. *British Journal of Psychology*. 2013 May; 104(2): 225–34

63. Carney DR, Cuddy AJC and Yap AJ. 'Power Posing: Brief Nonverbal Displays Affect Neuroendocrine Levels And Risk Tolerance.' *Psychological Science*. 2010 Oct; 21(10): 1363–8

64. Virtanen M et al. 'Long Working Hours and Alcohol Use: Systematic Review and Meta-Analysis Of Published Studies And Unpublished Individual Participant Data.' *British Medical Journal*. 2015 Jan 13; 350: g7772

65. Stoeber J and Janssen DP. 'Perfectionism and Coping With Daily Failures: Positive Reframing Helps Achieve Satisfaction at the End of the Day.' *Anxiety, Stress and Coping.* 2011 Oct; 24(5): 477–97

66. Research trials for the Aromacology Patch Company Ltd carried out by St George's Hospital London. Presented at the International Congress of Dietetics in Edinburgh 2000

67. Kemps E and Tiggemann M. 'A Cognitive Experimental Approach to Understanding and Reducing Food Cravings.' *Current Directions in Psychological Science.* 2010 April; 19 (2): 86–90

68. Goetz T et al. 'Types of Boredom: An Experience Sampling Approach.' *Motivation and Emotion.* 2014 June; 38 (3): 401–19

69. Brody S, Preut R, Schommer K and Schürmeyer TH. 'A Randomized Controlled Trial of High Dose Ascorbic Acid for Reduction of Blood Pressure, Cortisol, and Subjective Responses to Psychological Stress.' *Psychopharmacology* (Berl). 2002 Jan; 159(3): 319–24

70. Bradbury J, Myers SP and Oliver C. 'An Adaptogenic Role for Omega-3 Fatty Acids in Stress; A Randomised Placebo Controlled Double Blind Intervention Study' (pilot) *Nutrition Journal.* 2004 Nov 28; 3: 20

71. Downer B., Jiang Y., Zanjani F., and Fardo D. 'Effects of Alcohol Consumption on Cognition and Regional Brain Volumes Among Older Adults.' *American Journal of Alzheimer's Disease and Other Dementias.* 2015 Jun; 30(4): 364–74

72. Gémes K et al. 'Light-to-Moderate Drinking and Incident Heart Failure – The Norwegian HUNT Study.' *International Journal of Cardiology.* 2016 Jan 15; 203: 553–60

73. Koppes LL, Dekker JM, Hendriks HF, Bouter LM and Heine RJ. 'Moderate Alcohol Consumption Lowers the Risk of Type 2 Diabetes: A Meta-Analysis of Prospective Observational Studies.' *Diabetes Care.* 2005 Mar; 28(3): 719–25

74. Marrone JA et al. 'Moderate Alcohol Intake Lowers Biochemical Markers of Bone Turnover in Postmenopausal Women.' *Menopause.* 2012 Sep: 19(9): 974–9

75. Hansel B et al. 'Relationship Between Alcohol Intake, Health and Social Status and Cardiovascular Risk Factors in the Urban

Paris-Ile-De-France Cohort: Is the Cardioprotective Action of Alcohol a Myth?' *European Journal of Clinical Nutrition.* 2010 Jun; 64(6): 561–8

76. Marczinski CA and Stamates AL. 'Artificial Sweeteners Versus Regular Mixers Increase Breath Alcohol Concentrations in Male and Female Social Drinkers.' *Alcoholism, Clinical and Experimental Research.* 2013 Apr; 37(4): 696–702

77. Marczinski CA. 'Can Energy Drinks Increase the Desire for More Alcohol?' *Advances in Nutrition.* 2015 Jan; 6(1): 96–101

78. Department of Health Press Release. 'English Drinkers Knock Back Double Shots At Home.' December 2009

79. Walker D, Smarandescu L and Wansink B. 'Half Full or Empty: Cues That Lead Wine Drinkers to Unintentionally Overpour.' *Substance Use & Misuse.* 2014 Feb; 49(3): 295–302

80. Attwood AS, Scott-Samuel NE, Stothart G and Munafó MR. 'Glass Shape Influences Consumption Rate for Alcoholic Beverages.' *PLoS One.* 2012; 7(8): e43007

81. Walker D, Smarandescu L and Wansink B. 'Half Full or Empty: Cues That Lead Wine Drinkers to Unintentionally Overpour.' *Substance Use & Misuse.* 2014 Feb; 49(3): 295–302

82. Oksanen A and Kokkonen H. 'Consumption of Wine with Meals and Subjective Well-being: A Finnish Population-Based Study.' *Alcohol and Alcoholism.* 2016 Nov; 51(6): 716–72

83. Toledo E et al. 'Mediterranean Diet and Invasive Breast Cancer Risk among Women at High Cardiovascular Risk in the PREDIMED Trial: A Randomized Clinical Trial.' *JAMA Internal Medicine.* 2015; 175(11): 1752–60

84. Bauer PW, Pivarnik JM, Feltz D, Paneth N and Womack CJ. 'Relationship of Past-Pregnancy Physical Activity and Self-efficacy With Current Physical Activity and Postpartum Weight Retention.' *American Journal of Lifestyle Medicine.* 2013 Sept; 8(1): 68–73

85. David ME and Haws KL. 'Saying "No" to Cake or "Yes" to Kale: Approach and Avoidance Strategies in Pursuit of Health Goals.' *Psychology and Marketing.* 2106 August; 33(8): 588–94

86. National Weight Control Registry Facts – www.nwcr.ws

87. Brouwer AM and Mosack, KE. 'Motivating Healthy Diet Behaviors: The Self-as-Doer Identity.' *Self and Identity*. 2015 May; 14 (6): 638–53

88. Health & Social Care Information Centre. Statistics on Smoking, England, 2016

89. Rose JE and Behm FM. 'Inhalation of vapor from black pepper extract reduces smoking withdrawal symptoms.' *Drug and Alcohol Dependence*. 1994 Feb; 34(3): 225–9

90. Glass TW and Maher CG. 'Physical activity reduces cigarette cravings.' *British Journal of Sports Medicine*. 2014 Aug; 48(16): 1263–4

91. Wetherill R, Jagannathan K, Hager N, Maron M and Franklin T. 'Influence of menstrual cycle phase on resting-state functional connectivity in naturally cycling, cigarette-dependent women.' *Biology of Sex Differences*. 2016 May 10; 7: 24

92. British Heart Foundation Physical Activity Statistics 2015

93. Ruby MB, Dunn EW, Perrino A, Gillis R and Viel S. 'The invisible benefits of exercise.' *Health Psychology*. 2011 Jan; 30(1): 67–74

94. JP Morgan Chase & Co. 'Paychecks, Paydays and the Online Platform Economy.' *Big Data on Income Volatility* February 2016

95. Mogilner C, Chance Z and Norton MI. 'Giving Time Gives You Time.' *Psychological Science*. 2012 Oct 1; 23(10): 1233–38

Index